LU ANN ADAY, Ph.D.
GRETCHEN V. FLEMING, Ph.D.
RONALD ANDERSEN, Ph.D.

# Access To Medical Care In The U.S.:

# Who Has It, Who Doesn't

**pluribus Press inc.**

University of Chicago, Center for Health Administration Studies

Continuing CHAS Research Series—No. 32

89 88 87 86 85        5 4 3 2 1


Library of Congress Catalog Card Number:
84-61463


International Standard Book Number:
0-931028-56-6


Pluribus Press, Inc., Division of Teach'em, Inc.
160 East Illinois Street
Chicago, Illinois 60611

Center for Health Administration Studies
University of Chicago
5720 South Woodlawn
Chicago, IL 60637


*Printed in the United States of America*

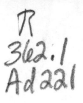

# Acknowledgements

The authors gratefully acknowledge the support provided by the Robert Wood Johnson Foundation (Princeton, New Jersey) for the analyses of the 1982 National Access Survey data. The project was entirely supported by grants from the Foundation.

We particularly appreciate the collegial support provided by the officers and staff of the Foundation—David Rogers, Bob Blendon, Linda Aiken and Catherine McCaslin—who worked with us on both the business and technical sides of the project.

Consultants Howard Freeman and Seymour Sudman provided valuable input into the overall design and execution of the study. We also appreciate the cooperation Lou Harris gave us in transmitting the data tape and in responding to questions regarding the form and content of the data itself.

The Center for Health Administration Studies (CHAS) has given us a supportive working environment. Special thanks go to numerous CHAS staff who worked with us in shaping and executing the analyses reported here: Sara

S. Loevy, Dr. P. H., Research Project Analyst, who helped supervise and carry out the cleaning of the data, constructed the algorithms for variables used in the analysis and wrote the variable definitions appendix (Appendix C) to the report; Christopher Lyttle, Programmer/ Analyst, who constructed the data file, designed and executed the cleaning and data imputation programs and coauthored Appendix D to the report; Martha J. Banks, Sampling Director, who consulted on the sample design for the study and developed the approaches for weighting and computing standard errors for the data described in Appendices A and B; Michael W. Cox, Programmer/ Analyst, who performed the majority of the analyses reported here; Ralph Bell, former CHAS Data Manager and Research Project Specialist, who provided guidance for the construction of the data file and the approach to the cleaning and data imputation procedures; Bob Cripe, Senior Programmer, who provided technical assistance in the analysis of the data and the preparation of the final report; Secretaries Annette Twells, Dorothy Frazier and Joyce Van Grondelle, who spent many hours inputting and editing the text, and to Research Assistants Margaret Aplington, Daryl Gernert and Anne Richard, who performed a variety of tasks to produce the manuscript that follows.

We hope you will find this book useful. As you can see, we have a number of individuals to thank for helping produce it, but we take full responsibility for its final form and content.

Lu Ann Aday, Ph.D.
Gretchen V. Fleming, Ph.D.
Ronald Andersen, Ph.D.
Chicago, Illinois
June 1984

# Table of Contents

Introduction
Policy issues
Ethical issues
Conceptual issues
Empirical issues

Measures of access and groups of interest
Potential access
Realized access: global indicators
Realized access: specific policy issues
Realized access: patient satisfaction
Summary: the picture of access in 1982

# Executive Summary

This book presents data from a 1982 National Survey of Access to Medical Care to inform the debate on the current "state-of-the-nation" with respect to access: i.e., whether the previous trends for the major indicators of access are continuing; which groups appear to have the greatest problems; and the severity of certain problems that might be exacerbated by the current political and economic climate, e.g., loss of insurance coverage or the financial or other barriers encountered in obtaining care for a family member with a serious illness.

In 1982, Lou Harris and Associates, with support from the Robert Wood Johnson Foundation (Princeton, New Jersey), conducted a telephone survey of a representative sample of 4,800 families in the United States, including a special oversample of 1,800 low-income families, to determine their current patterns of access to medical care and any special problems they had encountered in obtaining care during the previous year. One random adult and one random child (if one was present in the family) were selected for intensive interviews, yielding a total of 6,610 individual interviews. We estimate the overall response rate to be 60 percent. Post-stratification weights were applied to the data to adjust for the under- or overrepresentation of certain groups in the sample.

The Harris survey was modeled in part on earlier CHAS national surveys, allowing some trend analyses as far back as 1953. While the methodology across studies is not always exactly the same, the stability of these measures over time and their comparability for the most part to national estimates from the National Center for Health Statistics (NCHS) provides an opportunity to monitor possible changes in equity of access during a critical period in the financing and delivery of health services in the United States.

Improvements in access to medical care for traditionally disadvantaged groups documented in earlier decades largely continued into the 1980s. The poor, minority groups and central city and farm residents mostly maintained or improved their earlier gains relative to the rest of the population with respect to having a usual source of care or using hospital, physician and preventive services. However, some problems remain for these disadvantaged groups. They are less likely to identify with a particular practitioner; are more likely to use an outpatient department or emergency room as a regular source of care, and are subjected to longer average waiting times to see a physician. The most disadvantaged groups on most measures of access are the uninsured and those without a regular source of care.

The examination of data about families who felt they needed care and did not get it points out two aspects of the access problem. Some people do not get care they feel they need for the range of health problems most families face. They often lack personal resources and are not covered by public programs that would enable them to obtain care. The reasons for their inability to secure services are sometimes transitory and reversible. Frequently we find the uninsured and the unemployed in this group.

Another, and probably smaller, group faces long-term access problems created by chronic illness. They may well have basic coverage from public or other sources. However, this basic coverage does not extend to their special long-term needs, and they do not have sufficient personal resources to make up the deficit. Groups especially in need of longer term support include poor minorities and those covered by public programs alone.

Mounting budget deficits and efforts to cut costs make health care programs vulnerable, particularly in the public sector. Access to medical care should be closely monitored as financing and delivery programs are altered or cut back. The costs of reduced access as well as the benefits of reduced spending must be fully specified to inform future health care planning. Particular attention should be given to those groups most likely to be affected by such changes.

# Tables and Figures

# Chapter 1

## An Overview of Current Access Issues

### Introduction

During the 1960s and 1970s major private and federal initiatives were launched to improve access to medical care for key target groups: the elderly, the poor, inner city and rural residents, for example. These initiatives included Medicare, Medicaid, neighborhood health centers, the National Health Service Corps (NHSC) and related programs. National data collected during that period to monitor the impact of these programs on the population's access to medical care showed substantial improvements for many traditionally disadvantaged groups (Aday, et al., 1980; NCHS, 1980). Simultaneously, however, the levels of federal and personal expenditures for health care services have continued to rise, and the funding sources for major federal initiatives have been threatened or reduced.

In response to the skyrocketing costs of care, major

1

Administration and Congressional policy proposals early in the 1980s have focused on innovative alternatives for limiting federal and personal health care expenditures. Critics of these proposals have raised questions about their potentially negative impact on favorable access trends for traditionally disadvantaged groups and about the diminished probability of resolving persisting inequities exacerbated by unemployment and associated economic conditions that have affected certain groups since the mid-1970s.

This book presents data from a 1982 National Survey of Access to Medical Care to inform the debate on the current "state-of-the-nation" with respect to access; whether the previous trends are continuing for the major GNP-type indicators of access; which groups appear to have the greatest problems; and the severity of certain problems that might be aggravated by the current political and economic climate, e.g., loss of insurance coverage or the financial or other barriers encountered in obtaining care for a family member with a serious illness.

In 1982, Lou Harris and Associates, with support from the Robert Wood Johnson Foundation (Princeton, New Jersey), conducted a telephone survey of a representative sample of 4,800 families in the United States, including a special oversample of 1,800 low-income families to determine their access to medical care and any special problems that they had encountered in obtaining care during the previous year (Lou Harris and Associates, 1982). One random adult and one random child (if one was present in the family) were selected for intensive interviews, yielding a total of 6,610 individual interviews. (A detailed description of the sample design and weighting procedures applied to the data are provided in Appendix A.)

This chapter considers the major policy proposals and their probable impact on access. Particular attention is given to the ethical implications of these proposals in the context of equity of access. The conceptual framework and empirical emphases to be applied in examining these issues are also introduced.

Chapter 2 presents the 1982 survey data for major traditional access indicators for key population subgroups and for the U.S. population as a whole. When available, national survey data from previous years are also presented to trace trends in major access indicators. This chapter provides a descriptive overview of the biggest problems with respect to frontline medical care access for key population subgroups of the greatest interest in health policy formulation, e.g., children, the elderly, inner city and rural residents, poor minorities and the unemployed and uninsured.

Chapter 3 is more analytic in focus. In this chapter, we draw on the descriptive between-group and over-time comparisons in Chapter 2 to identify key access indicators and subgroups in an effort to understand more fully the reasons for any observed inequities. Applying our equity of access framework developed in Chapter 1 and multivariate modeling, we attempt to determine the extent to which equitable need-related factors; inequitable population attributes not easily manipulated by health policy (e.g., income or racial correlates), and mutable policy relevant factors (e.g., insurance coverage, linkages with a regular source of care) contribute to any observed access differences. These analyses should serve to inform policymakers and other interested providers and consumers about 1) what can (and perhaps what cannot) be changed in the effort to alter existing inequities and 2) the extent to which policies to reduce services or benefits might reintroduce or exacerbate inequities.

Chapter 4 examines findings on questions that were asked about special access problems encountered by U.S.

families and individuals. These access questions were introduced in the 1982 study and therefore are not available on previous national surveys. They do, however, permit closer examination of potential and realized access problems which may confront special subgroups of people in periods of economic recession and fiscal austerity such as those which have characterized the 1980s to date. These problems include increased difficulty in obtaining care; losing insurance coverage or being refused care for financial reasons; or experiencing major financial problems as a result of a serious illness in the family.

In the final chapter we attempt to project future equity of access in the context of current and proposed health policy options. This chapter attempts to integrate and interpret what we have learned from previous access studies, what the most current findings suggest to deal with remaining problems and the kind of information that should be routinely collected to monitor the state of the nation's health with respect to the system goal of equity of access.

The findings to be presented represent the most current national data available to address these questions. In addition, they provide highly relevant new indicators for monitoring current access and fine-tuning the focus on problems of particular relevance in the '80s. In initially designing the study, we made an effort to develop indicators that could be compared with previous national studies of access conducted by the Center for Health Administration Studies (CHAS), The University of Chicago and the National Center for Health Statistics (NCHS). There were major changes in a number of key items in the 1982 NCHS-Health Interview Survey (HIS), which will make over-time comparisons using that data more problematic (Givens and Moss, 1981). Hence, these 1982 Harris survey data are of particular interest because they allow a timely monitoring of developing changes in the American health care system. This is the kind of information that policymakers need to make informed and equitable choices. The remainder of this chapter reviews the nature and implications of the choices confronting policymakers, and, ultimately, health care providers and the American public.

## Policy issues

Expenditures for health care resources and services have increased dramatically over the past 20 years. In the mid-1960s, the period in which major federal financing initiatives in health care were introduced, Americans spent $42 billion — six percent of the Gross National Product (GNP) — on health care. Approximately 26 percent of all national health expenditures were from public funds. By 1981 aggregate expenditures for health increased sixfold to $287 billion, or 9.8 percent of the nation's GNP in 1981. The federal share of those dollars had increased by almost two-thirds to 43 percent (Waldo and Gibson, 1982). In 1984, 10.5 percent of the nation's GNP is estimated to be spent on health.

These increased expenditures were accompanied by recognition that fewer resources are, in fact, available to both the public and private sectors to finance health care programs in the 1980s (Blendon, et al., 1981). There is evidence, for example, that the Hospital Insurance Trust Fund that provides funds for the Medicare program may well be bankrupt by the end of the 1980s unless new ways can be found to lower the rate of expenditures under this program (Congressional Budget Office, 1983).

The assumption in the 1960s was that adequate resources were available to assure access to care for all Americans. The introduction of a multiplicity of financing and organizationally-oriented programs during this period reflected this confidence. In the 1970s the finitude of resources came to be recognized; current evidence points to more cutbacks, rather than introduction of costly new programs in the 1980s. This evidence also implies that cost containment, rather than access, will be the major health policy "bandwagon" in the decade ahead (Hitt and Harristhal, 1980; Weiner, 1980).

The response to these cost-containment concerns has produced a variety of proposals for dealing with the increasing cost of care. "Pro-competition" has been a major theme in many of the policy options suggested for consideration (Langwell and Moore, 1982). The Reagan Administration has provided considerable support for this objective, in addition to encouraging cutbacks in the Medicare and Medicaid programs; decentralizing more health care services to the states through the block grant concept; and arguing for the states to take over the Medicaid program itself (Enright, 1982; Iglehart, 1981).

Major theorists for the pro-competition concept have included Alain Enthoven and Clark Havighurst, among others. Enthoven has argued for a Consumer Choice Health Plan (CCHP) with the following elements: 1) a multiple choice option in which consumers would be offered the opportunity each year to enroll in any qualified plan available in their area; 2) a fixed-dollar subsidy, which would promote cost consciousness requiring the person who chose a more costly health plan to pay more; 3) application of the same rules governing premium-setting, minimum benefit packages, catastrophic protection and so on to all health plans to prevent preferred-risk selection or excessive costs for high-risk enrollees, and 4) organization of physicians into competing economic units, and tying the premium charged by each plan to the ability of its associated physicians to contain costs. The CCHP would also limit the tax-free employer contributions to health benefits, so that employees would become more directly aware of the actual costs of purchasing those benefits (Enthoven, 1980; 1981).

Similarly, Havighurst has argued for a national agenda of encouraging maximum competition for the business of informed consumers among providers of care. This would be supported by vigorous federal government enforcement of antitrust laws against collusion by providers and by elimination of cost-inefficient tax incentives. The needs of the poor and uninsurable would, he argues, be met through direct public subsidies, actuarially adjusted tax credits and other approaches that would not diminish competition and efficiency (Havighurst, 1982).

An important element of this pro-competition strategy is the development of a variety of providers which would compete successfully with each other. Health Maintenance Organizations (HMOs) are one form of organization which integrates both the service delivery and financing components that have been credited with inducing more cost-efficient behavior on the part of the providers and consumers of care (Luft, 1981). Preferred Provider Organizations (PPOs) are another developing modality in which insurance companies might, for example, catalyze the formation of a panel of providers to facilitate the containment of the costs of care they provide to consumers enrolled with them through the insuring companies (Egdahl, 1981).

Some states are beginning to explicitly implement these pro-competition strategies. California, for example, enacted legislation to intensify competition among hospitals and physicians in an effort to deal with a projected $2 billion deficit in its state budget, recurrent cost overruns in the MediCal (Medicaid) program and a 17.9 percent increase in hospital costs in 1981. The legislation authorized both the government and private insurance companies to negotiate prepaid contracts with hospitals and providers as a mechanism for containing health care costs (Melia, et al., 1983). Similar initiatives are underway in Arizona in the Arizona Health Care Cost Containment Experiment. In this initiative the state is, for the first time, introducing a Medicaid-type program for the medically indigent in which providers can enter into contracts with county governments to provide services to eligible beneficiaries.

Competition in the hospital sector was catalyzed in September 1982 when Congress enacted a major change in the method of reimbursing hospitals for services provided through Medicare. The Tax Equity and Fiscal Responsibility Act of 1982 (TEFRA) directed the Department of Health and Human Services (DHHS) to develop a prospective payment formula that, when implemented, would in effect impose a spending ceiling on Medicare for hospital services (Iglehart, 1982b). This mechanism will replace the former "reasonable" cost reimbursement policy with one that requires Medicare to establish prices in advance on a cost-per-case basis, using as a measure 467 categories of diagnosis-related groups (DRGs). The clear intent of the new law is, Iglehart argues, "to compel hospitals through a new set of economic incentives, to change their institutional behavior and in turn persuade physicians to husband their resources more judiciously" (Iglehart, 1983: 1430).

Another response to the increasingly evident cost constraints on costly inpatient care is to encourage the substitution of ambulatory for inpatient services. For example, ambulatory surgery has become a more common cost-containment alternative (Berk and Chalmers, 1981; Detmer, 1981; Marks, et al., 1980). Further, physicians, responding to increasingly-felt competition from other physicians and institutional providers, are themselves becoming more involved in the business of establishing their own freestandin᷉g emergi-care and birthing centers (Friedman, 1982).

There are critics of the pro-competition strategies and their probable impact whose voices are being heard in the current policy debates as well. McNerney, for example, has argued that a balance between the competition and regulation strategies, combined with an emphasis on preventive services and health education, would effect the best long-term improvement in health status and, ultimately, reduced health care costs due to illness (McNerney, 1980).

Others argue that the competitive proposals will, in fact, not yield the desired cost containment objectives or, even worse, produce a two-tiered system of care in which those less able to pay have poor access and quality of services (Ginzberg, 1980; 1983). For example, Luft presents evidence that increased competition may improve efficiency, but it may also increase emphasis by HMOs and other insurers on selective marketing, cost shifting, experience rating and other mechanisms that directly and adversely affect the poor, the elderly and the seriously ill (Luft, 1982). Mechanic, too, argues that cuts most often occur at the point of "least political resistance"—i.e., the poor, the old and the chronically ill (Mechanic, 1981). Iglehart presents data which shows that Reagan's massive tax reductions and cuts in social welfare programs in 1981 and 1982 resulted in an income redistribution least favorable to the poor and lower-middle-income groups, while middle-income groups "held their own, and virtually all real benefits accrued to the well-off" (Iglehart, 1982a: 838).

Obsession with cost may increasingly lead to the "corporate rationalization" of health care as well (Pollitt,

1982) and the associated fragmentation of health and welfare services (Snoke, 1982). Iglehart further argues that the prospective payment of hospitals may give these institutions a new incentive to "underserve patients" (Igelhart, 1983: 1430) and to perhaps compromise the quantity or quality of care rendered to publicly financed beneficiaries in particular.

There is substantial evidence from both Canada (Beck and Horne, 1980) and the Rand Health Insurance Experiment in the United States (Fein, 1981; Newhouse, et al., 1981; 1982) that increased cost sharing does indeed lead to reduction in services for those who have to pay more out-of-pocket for care. Whether these reductions also ultimately influence health status is still being evaluated (Brook, et al., 1983).

## Ethical issues

If, as suggested, cost containment strategies compromise the equity of access to medical services for certain groups, then ethical issues surrounding this expressed equity goal become important in informed consideration of these alternatives.

In the 1980s emphasis on costs has reduced the salience of the equity of access objective (Aday and Andersen, 1981; Ginzberg, 1978; President's Commission, 1983). There is evidence that considerable progress has been made since the mid-1960s in reducing access differentials for traditionally disadvantaged groups (Aday, et al., 1980). A number of programs, which are currently being considered for reductions or have already been substantially reduced in scope as a result of Administrative and Congressional proposals, are credited with contributing to these successes: for example, Medicaid (Rogers, et al., 1982); the Early Periodic Screening, Diagnostic and

Treatment Program (Foltz, 1982), and the Neighborhood/ Community Health Center Program (Freeman, et al., 1982; Goldman and Grossman, 1982; Okada and Wan, 1980).

Concern is expressed that eliminating these programs or increasing the financial burden on lower- or middle-income families through cost sharing or tighter eligibility requirements may, in fact, reverse the favorable trends observed to date (Aday and Andersen, 1981).

Others point out that substantial inequities continue to exist for certain groups. Low-income children, even those covered by Medicaid, continue to have fewer physician and dental contacts and poorer health, and are more likely to be seen by public or institutional, rather than private, providers (Gortmaker, 1981; Kovar, 1982; Orr and Miller, 1981). Though mean physician visit rates are converging for high- and low-income adults, adjustments for health status suggest that, relative to their need, lower-income individuals are still less likely to see a physician than are those with higher incomes (Davis, et al., 1981; Kleinman, et al., 1981).

The uninsured and the poor who "slip through the cracks" of existing public insurance programs are particularly less likely to have seen a doctor and used hospital services than those with insurance. These differences are larger than health status differentials alone would indicate (Davis and Rowland, 1983; Wilensky and Berk, 1982). The number of uninsured and the proportion of poor with diminished purchasing power are apt to increase, rather than to decrease, as a result of many of the program reductions and cost-sharing proposals being considered or enacted by Congress and the Administration. As a result, there are fears that these changes may not only reverse favorable trends of the past but exacerbate the inequities that do remain.

Trying to arrive at "ethical" methods to achieve equity of access in the context of the equally important need to contain the ever-increasing costs of care is not guided by clearly specified criteria or well-articulated operational definitions of "what is right." The President's Commission for the Study of Ethical Problems in Medicine and Biomedical and Behavioral Research recently released a report which maintains that "society has a moral obligation to ensure that everyone has access to adequate care without being subject to excessive burdens" (President's Commission, I, 1983: 22). The keystone of the Commission's approach to assessing equity of access is the concept of "adequate care" based on professionally-derived judgments, average current use levels, particular minimum service requirements and overall summary judgments of adequacy. Neither the adequacy criterion, nor other standards of appropriateness, are easily applied to difficult resource allocation decisions that involve a variety of constituencies and (perhaps) competing goals such as the current access vs cost-containment considerations (President's Commission, III, 1983).

Some critics argue that equity of access to health care may not be an appropriate broad societal goal (Daniels, 1982; Guttman, 1981). Data from England suggest that other more general social conditions (such as social class, education, housing and race) may have more bearing on persistent inequities in health and health care than do the factors policymakers or system planners can directly alter (Gray, 1982; Hollingsworth, 1981).

Decisions about the allocation of resources to equity of access versus cost containment objectives are ultimately political ones (Vladeck, 1981). Such choices should, however, be made in the context of the best available information on the probable impact of those choices (Breslow, 1981; Rice, 1981). Our framework for analyzing the equity of access objective and the progress of the U.S. health care system toward that goal is discussed in the following section to provide an informed basis for considering competing political options.

## Conceptual issues

The basic framework for considering the access concept was first introduced by the authors in 1975 (Aday and Andersen, 1975) (See Figure 1.1). It built upon and elaborated a behavioral model of determinants of families' utilization of health services (Andersen, 1968). The framework was applied directly in the collection and analyses of data for a national survey of access to medical care conducted in 1976 (Aday, et al., 1980) and in subsequent community-survey based evaluations of the access impact of innovative health care programs: the Robert Wood Johnson Foundation-supported Community Hospital Program (CHP) (Aday, et al., 1984) and the Health Care Financing Administration (HCFA)-supported Municipal Health Services Program (MHSP) evaluation (Andersen, et al., 1982). Many of the same indicators applied in these studies were also included in the 1982 access survey to enhance the comparability between data sources.

According to our framework, access may be defined as those dimensions which describe the potential and actual entry of a given population group to the health care delivery system. The probability of an individual's entry into the health care system is influenced by the structure of the delivery system itself (the availability and organization of health care resources) and the nature of the wants, resources and needs that potential consumers may bring to the care-seeking process. The realization of the objective of entry is reflected in a population's reported rates of utilization and in the subjective evaluations of the care its members eventually obtain.

## FIGURE 1.1  Framework for the Study of Access

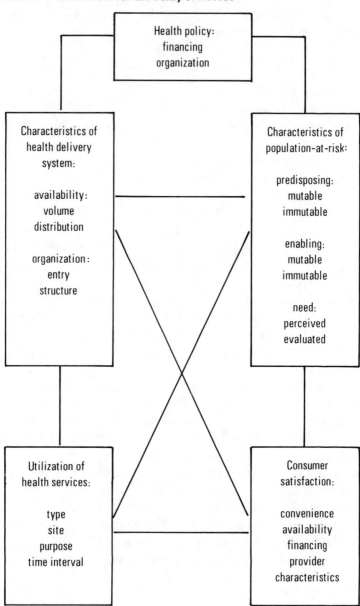

Whether one has a regular source of medical care, the distance one has to travel to care, the type of insurance coverage one has, and one's total annual income can affect one's ability to obtain wanted or needed care, as well as how satisfactory the process of care-seeking will be. Utilization rates and satisfaction scores, however, describe the actual impact of these and a variety of other determinants. These more immediate outcomes, rather than changes in health status, are taken as the end points of the access model because a variety of factors other than contact with the health care system per se can affect health status (hereditary, nutritional and environmental influences, for example) and because access is generally assumed to imply right of entry to the system, regardless of ultimate changes in the health status of the population.

Since our framework was introduced, other researchers have also described and presented data on their preferred approaches to the definition and measurement of access (Davis and Reynolds, 1975; Hulka, 1978; Lewis, et al., 1976; Penchansky and Thomas, 1981; Shortell, et al., 1977; Sloan and Bentkover, 1979). Many of the elements just described in connection with our framework are also used by these access researchers, e.g., the availability of medical resources in an area, the convenience of these services to potential consumers and how service utilization rates relative to need vary for different groups.

In a presentation on the equity of access goal to the President's Commission for the Study of Ethical Problems in Medical Care which was subsequently published in a special supplement to *Medical Care,* we elaborated the various concepts of equity that would be operationalized with the framework (Aday and Andersen, 1981; President's Commission, III, 1983). We have particularly emphasized the criterion for equity of access that maintains that it exists when services are distributed on the basis of people's need for them. Inequity exists, on the other hand, when services are distributed on the basis of personal characteristics such as race, family income or place of residence rather than need.*

This framework will serve to guide the analyses that follow, particularly in Chapter 3, to determine the relative importance of equitable and inequitable factors in explaining current access outcomes.

Some of the empirical issues of particular relevance in the analyses are discussed in the following section.

## Empirical issues

To the extent possible, findings of the current study will be compared with earlier studies to better establish possible trends in access over time. Examining these trends is one way of gauging the probable impact of policy and program alternatives on the access of target groups most directly affected by these initiatives (e.g., the poor, the elderly, etc.).

Caution should be exercised in making such comparisons, however. The questions are not always identical in the respective studies because changes in the mode of interview (from face-to-face to telephone, for example) required compromises, as well as for a variety of other reasons. Differences in the mode of data collection (in-person or by phone) could affect the comparability of estimates. (The previous studies to be compared here were all in-person, whereas the 1982 study was by phone.) Dif-

---

* Operational definitions used in expressing the equity of access objective in terms of use relative to need, especially the use disability ratio, have been criticized in the literature. (See a discussion on pages 185–188 of Aday, et al., 1980 and more recently in Marcus and Stone, 1982 and Yergan, et al., 1981.)

ferent sample designs or variant response rates—particularly variable subgroup non-response rates—could affect the comparability of the universe in fact represented by different studies. Some estimates may depart considerably from other relatively current and comparable sources, giving rise to concerns about unknown biases that may exist in the data. (This is, in fact, true for several key estimates in the 1982 data, and is discussed in more detail in Chapter 2 and the accompanying appendices.)

The following analyses focus on 1) certain population subgroups for whom there have been or are currently concerns about equity, and 2) policy-relevant issues likely to have the greatest impact on access and be most amenable to public policy changes.

Subgroups of special interest when the equity of access objective is considered are children and the elderly (Kovar, 1982; Estes, 1982); racial minorities (Wolinsky, 1982); low-income individuals (Kleinman, et al., 1981; Newacheck, et al., 1980); inner city and rural residents (Okada and Wan, 1980; Rosenblatt and Moscovice, 1982) and the unemployed and uninsured.

Particular emphasis will be placed on examining the characteristics of the organization and financing of services from the consumer point of view. Access and convenience have been found to vary considerably according to whether people have a regular source of care and the characteristics of this regular provider (Dutton and Silber, 1980; Kasper and Barrish, 1982; Kasper and Berk, 1981; Master, et al., 1980; Sawyer, 1982; Wolinsky and Marder, 1982). Insurance coverage and its availability all or part of the year also significantly affect realized access to care—in particular rates of physician and hospital utilization (Davis, et al., 1981; Davis and Rowland, 1983; Kasper, et al., 1980; Wilensky and Berk, 1982). This financing aspect of access is particularly important in the context of the health policy debate described earlier and the real tradeoffs that arise in trying to realize both access and cost-containment objectives.

The following analyses present data on both traditional indicators of potential and realized access to care and new measures relevant to the particular political and economic environment of the 1980s.

# Chapter 2

## The National Picture of Access

Six years separated the last national survey conducted expressly to measure access to medical care and the 1982 study of access reported here (See Aday, et al., 1980). As noted in Chapter 1, a number of changes occurred on the national scene during that time, including 1) heightened sensitivity to the ever-increasing percentage of the Gross National Product (GNP) attributable to health care costs; 2) a change in national policy which included major cutbacks in expenditures for publicly funded medical programs, and 3) a recession that saw unemployment rise to levels higher than any since the 1930s.

This chapter will present basic descriptive data on key parameters of access for the first time since these changes have taken place. In addition, we will discuss changes that may have occurred in those indicators for which we have comparable (or at least similar) data from earlier time periods. Finally, this chapter will lay the groundwork for more probing analyses of the current profile of access which will be presented in the chapters that follow.

## Measures of access and groups of interest

Our framework for access is multidimensional (see Chapter 1). Therefore, we will present data on a number of measures of access. Initially, we may describe all of these measures as falling into one of two types: "potential" and "realized" measures of access. "Potential" access refers to those indicators that describe the process of obtaining medical care. They may be viewed as structural features of the system that help determine whether people obtain care, as well as the type and quality of that care. "Realized" access describes the services actually received in terms of units of care, e.g., doctor visits, as well as subjective perceptions of care received, e.g., patient satisfaction with the services (Aday, et al., 1980: 30–32). Measures of potential access that will be examined here will include the existence of a regular source of care, characteristics of that source and average waiting time in a doctor's office.

Measures of realized access will be both objective and subjective. Objective measures might be described as two kinds. The first comprises those which assess the "global" picture in ways analogous to how the GNP measures the economy. Such measures would include percentage of people who have seen a physician and the average number of visits to a doctor. The second consists of more specific, policy-relevant measures of use: e.g., certain preventive services and the proportion of emergency room visits. Subjective measures include levels of patient dissatisfaction with aspects of the care received during the respondent's most recent medical visit.

Most of the access measures in this and subsequent chapters will be presented for key population subgroups. These groups have been chosen according to several criteria. Some of these criteria represent different levels of need, e.g., age. Others are characteristics which we have traditionally monitored because they have been shown to have a significant bearing on inequities in access in the past, e.g., race and poverty level.

In this report we have added breakdowns of the population which we feel are relevant, given the economic and political climate of the 1980s. These include employment status and insurance coverage. In addition, although we show a breakdown by ethnic group as well as one by income, we also present a four-part categorization of the population by race and poverty level, as we have learned that there can be a significant interaction between these two variables (Aday, et al., 1980).

## Potential access

Past studies have shown that having a regular source of care, a place one usually goes or which is identified as one's own source, is an important predictor not only of service utilization but also of satisfaction with what one gets (Aday, et al., 1980; Aday and Andersen, 1975). Moreover, having a regular source of care often equates with greater continuity of care, generally considered desirable because it enhances in general the quality of care received (Alpert, et al., 1970; Becker, et al., 1974; Breslau, 1982; Breslau and Mortimer, 1981; Breslau and Reeb, 1975; Freeborn and Greenlick, 1973; Heagarty, et al., 1970; Mindlin and Densen, 1969; Starfield, et al., 1976). Among other reasons, continuity of care and having a regular source are associated with compliance to prescribed treatment (Becker, et al., 1972), an essential ingredient of quality care.

However, having a regular source does not assure per se that all outcomes will be positive. The kind of source may also be critical in obtaining continuous care. Having a hospital outpatient department or emergency room as a regular source is considered inappropriate for the population in general, not only because it may be associated with less continuous care than a private doctor's office (CHAS, 1982; Chapter VI), but also because it generally provides care that is less satisfying to the patient and more costly (Aday, et al., 1980; CHAS, 1982: Chapters VII, X). Moreover, we have found in earlier work that there is a significant distinction between those whose source is the same doctor and those who go to one place for care but do not see one particular doctor there. In many ways, the latter group appears more similar to those with no source than to those with a physician (or other practitioner) that they can name. For instance, those who do not name a physician show about the same levels of dissatisfaction with care as those who have no regular source (Aday, et al., 1980: Chapter 4).

Table 2.1 shows the percent who reported having a particular doctor as a regular source of care, the percent who reported having a regular source but not a particular doctor, and the percent who did not have a regular source in 1982. Where the data are comparable, we have also presented the 1976 and 1970 figures. First of all, if we focus on the third set of columns, it appears that the percent without a regular source of care has held steady over this 13-year period. For 1982 it was 11 percent, compared to 12 percent and 11 percent for 1976 and 1970, respectively. In fact, when we look at the patterns for specific groups, it appears that there have been very small changes, if any, these last six years.

The main difference for most subgroups of the population is that fewer people are reporting no regular source of care. Among ethnic groups, Blacks are still less likely than Whites to have a regular source of care. This was also the case in 1976, when 15 percent of the "Black" group reported having no regular source and in 1970, when 16 percent of Blacks were in this category. Those in families with an unemployed main wage earner are also less likely to cite a regular source than are the employed and those with a main wage earner not in the labor force (which includes a large segment of retired people who, being older and more often ill, are more likely than average to have a customary point of entry into the system). The percent of those not employed without a regular source of care has not increased since 1976 (of course there are more unemployed), although there was a decrease of six percentage points between 1970 and 1976 for this group. The group that stands out most dramatically is the uninsured, with 22 percent reporting no regular source of care. This percentage has changed little if at all since 1976.

Of some interest is the middle set of columns in this table. Whereas the percent with no source of care may have diminished slightly, the number reporting a specific place but no particular doctor seems to have grown slightly but consistently larger for most groups since 1976. This is particularly noticeable for the 55 to 64 year-old group, rural farm dwellers and the uninsured. We will speculate on the possible reasons for this slight change in our summary at the end of the chapter. The situation may be different for Blacks, who were still somewhat more likely than Whites in particular to report no particular doctor in 1982. The group overall most likely to report no particular doctor is indicated by a measure of income (poverty level) by race (White versus nonwhite). Twenty-four percent of the nonwhite poor group report a regular source with no particular doctor.

Finally, the first column enables us to compare groups in 1982 and over time in terms of the optimal situation, having one doctor as a regular source of care. It is clear that among the groups we report for 1982, Blacks are the ethnic group least likely to have a particular doctor. Sixty-seven percent of Blacks have a particular doctor compared to 79 percent of the Whites—a full 12 percentage points less. The poor nonwhite group is even less apt to have a particular doctor; only 64 percent report they do. The trend for Blacks is, however, to have a particular doctor. The most comparable data for 1976 are for the nonwhites. At that time 62 percent of them reported a particular doctor, compared to the 67 percent in 1982. In 1976 only 50 percent of the urban nonwhite poor could name a regular doctor (data not shown), compared to 64 percent of the nonwhite poor now (Aday, et al., 1980: 51). Although part of this difference may be attributable to differences in methodology between the two studies (e.g., the more recent one was a telephone study, the earlier one, household), the differences are of such magnitude, for the poverty level and race comparisons in particular, that we may conclude that the situation has probably improved for this group. The Black population still is less well off than other segments of the population in 1982 according to this measure, however. Also of note is the relatively lower percentage of the unemployed with a particular doctor (70 percent versus 77 percent for the employed) and the very low percent (59 percent) of the uninsured who can name a regular doctor.

Another way of understanding the different usual sources of care for the U.S. population is to look at the location of these sources. The first column in Table 2.2 shows these data for the 89 percent of the population that did report a regular source. The overwhelming majority of this group, 83 percent, report a doctor's office (or private clinic). The next largest group goes to a hospital outpatient department (this group also includes those who mentioned a hospital but did not specify the type of unit).

Four percent report a government clinic, which includes "neighborhood" and public health clinics as well as other clinics that receive support primarily through government sources. Only two percent regularly go to an emergency room, and four percent are distributed among other types of clinics.

The second column in Table 2.2 presents similar data for the group who said they did not have a regular source of care but could mention a place they "would go" if they needed care. Seven percent of the 11 percent without a regular source of care responded to this question. Again, the overwhelming majority—76 percent—cited a doctor's office or private clinic. The rest were distributed similarly to those with a regular source, with slightly higher percentages mentioning the more commonly used sources.

A key access issue in the 1980s is the use of the hospital outpatient department and emergency room for primary care, because of the high unit cost of hospital-based care. Reporting such a source as a regular source of care is one indicator of the probability of use of that service. Table 2.3 shows the percent of those in each population group with a regular source of care that reports the hospital as their source (i.e., either outpatient department or emergency room). The percent increases with age, with the oldest group most likely to report this source. It is also larger for the central city than for other SMSA populations, and for the rural farm over other rural or small urban groups. There is an inverse relationship between income and the probability of having a hospital as a regular source of care. The hospital is more likely to be used by low-income people. Not surprisingly, nonwhite groups are more apt to report using a hospital outpatient department or emergency room than is the White majority. Being unemployed also is related to a higher probability of using this source as is having insurance through public programs (mostly Medicare and Medicaid) or being uninsured. The nonwhite poor are most likely to report using a hospital outpatient department or emergency room.

Another measure of potential access which significantly affects realized access measures is waiting time in the doctor's office. Not only is it a measure of the general efficiency of care from the patient's point of view, but, as will be shown later, it constitutes one of the aspects of medical care most often criticized by the patient.

Table 2.4 presents information on the length of time people waited to see the doctor at their last medical visit during the recall period for the 1982 study (if it was within a year of the interview date). Overall, 83 percent did not wait more than 30 minutes to see the doctor, whereas 12 percent waited between 30 and 60 minutes, and another 5 percent waited over 60 minutes. Among subgroups of the population, it is clear that ethnic minorities—Hispanics and Blacks—were more apt to wait a long time than the White majority. If poor, they were even more likely to wait a long time. Twenty-two percent of poor Whites waited over thirty minutes to see the doctor (15 percent plus 7 percent) compared to 14 percent of nonpoor Whites. Twenty-eight percent of poor nonwhites waited over thirty minutes to see the doctor, compared with 19 percent of nonpoor nonwhites. In addition, the unemployed were more apt to wait than those who were employed or not in the labor force, and the uninsured were substantially more apt to wait over thirty minutes than were those with some type of coverage.

## Realized access: global indicators

These indicators of access are important because they measure the fact that people actually got into the system and obtained specific services. In addition, they appear often in the research literature; therefore, national norms are oftentimes available for comparison. The measures are: the percent contacting the physician during the year recall period; the mean number of doctor visits for those contacting the physician; the percent hospitalized in·a year; the mean number of hospital admissions, and the mean number of nights in the hospital.

Table 2.5 presents data on the percent contacting the physician. Overall, this figure is 81 percent of the national population for 1982. This is a substantially higher figure than the 76 percent reported for 1976. The definition of a doctor contact was changed for the 1982 study, however, and the evidence is quite clear that this methodological change led to the higher estimates. The National Center for Health Statistics (NCHS) monitors this indicator annually. NCHS' 1981 data show that the percent seeing the doctor in that year was 74.3, slightly lower than the 74.9 reported for 1980 and the 75.1 for 1979 (NCHS, 1982a). The following change was made in the question eliciting doctor contact information: in 1982 we explicitly asked people to include visits in which "a nurse or other medical person on the doctor's staff" was seen instead of the doctor. In the 1976 version of the question, this cue was omitted. In addition, in 1982 two screener questions were asked to elicit doctor contacts in the previous year. Individuals who did not report having seen a doctor in the previous 12 months were asked the second probe about someone on the doctor's staff, as well as the doctor.

Table 2.5 shows similar rank ordering of age groups on this indicator across the 24 years for which we have these data, with the youngest group, under six, most likely to see a doctor; a dip in percentage for the older children, and a rise in general for the adult groups. Among the adults, the 35 to 54-year-olds are least likely to see the doctor. Rural people, especially those living on farms, are still less likely to see a doctor than are those living in urban areas. In 1982 race and employment status differences are not significant. In 1976 and 1970 the unemployed were only slightly less apt to contact the doctor than the employed. The high doctor contact rate in 1982 for those not in the labor force is probably due to the high percentage of elderly retired persons in this group. This rate appears to have increased relative to the rate for the employed majority over the years. There has been substantial change in the doctor contact rate for Blacks since 1970, when they were much less apt to see a physician in the year than were Whites. The poor are slightly less likely to see a doctor in the course of a year than are the nonpoor. The group that stands out as substantially less likely to see a doctor than others is the uninsured. This appears to be a stable pattern, at least since 1976.

Table 2.6 shows the mean number of physician visits during the year for those who reported a doctor contact. Data for 1976 are again shown, although comparisons between 1982 and 1976 are affected by the change in methodology reported above, as are the contact measures. The overall mean number of doctor visits for those seeing the doctor in 1982 was 6.1. The means are higher for adult age groups than for children. The difference between the rural farm group and the other residence groups does not appear as high as in 1976, either because of a change in patterns of care or the inclusion of visits with other medical personnel. The pattern of fewer doctor visits for those with higher incomes is still evident, due in part to higher illness levels among the poor (a situation which will be explored further in Chapter 3). The difference in average number of visits for Blacks and Whites is not significant. Individuals in families where the main wage earner was unemployed in 1982 seem to have a higher average number of visits than those where the main wage earner is employed, but the differences, again, are not significant. They were more substantial in 1976. It could be that these differences reflect a difference in health status; this will be examined further for the 1982 data in Chapter 3. Those not in the labor force have the highest level of doctor visits; again, this is due to the high percentage of retired people in this group.

The group which has the highest average number of visits is the publicly insured group (mostly Medicaid or Medicare). This may be due in part to its higher relative need. It may also be a function of a more fragmented, discontinuous profile of followup care for the poor and publicly insured. The public and private group is dominated by Medicare beneficiaries who have a supplemental private policy, and therefore their relatively high level of use may be partly an age and illness effect. The race-by-poverty-level breakdown demonstrates a higher level of use by the poor even more clearly than the income distribution. The hypotheses suggested here about the sources of some of these differences will be explored later in Chapter 3.

Table 2.7 compares 1982 data on physician utilization and NCHS distributions for 1980. Here the United States population is divided into categories, based on distributions of the number of doctor visits in the course of a year. The first column presents an estimate of the total population in the category. The next ten columns may be viewed as pairs, the first in each pair displaying the percentage of the population in that group according to NCHS data and the second the percentage derived from the 1982 Access Study. It is clear from this table that the Access Study percentages for almost every category shown for visits equal to "none" and visits equal to "1" are smaller than the NCHS statistics, whereas for the two largest amount of visits, "5–12" and "13 or more," the access study yielded larger percentages of the population than did the NCHS data (NCHS, 1983: 34).

Our conclusion that the higher average doctor contact rate and higher average numbers of visits reported in the 1982 Access Study resulted from the additional probes is supported by an NCHS methodological study. The NCHS study showed that a substantially higher average number of physician visits was reported by a randomly selected subgroup of its U.S. national sample who were asked to include in their responses visits to specific physician specialists (visits often believed to be forgotten by respondents) as well as "visits to a nurse or anyone else working with or for a medical doctor" (Givens and Moss, 1981). However, NCHS has also changed this question in its annual survey specifically to cue respondents to include these practitioners. Despite the lack of comparability between these current surveys and earlier work, it seems important to include this cue in light of the growing use of nurse practitioners in recent years and the frequency with which ancillary personnel may be providing primary care in larger group practices, especially HMOs (Luft, 1981).

Another critical area of utilization is inpatient care, because it is the primary component of high health care costs. Table 2.8 shows the percent hospitalized during the recall period for the 1982 study and the comparison data for 1976. The total percent hospitalized in the course of a year has not significantly changed. In addition, percentages remain similar for the subgroups for which we have data. Not surprisingly those categories that include the highest percentages of elderly show the highest percent hospitalized in the course of a year. As in earlier times, the poor are a little more apt to be hospitalized in the course of a year than are the nonpoor.

Table 2.9 elaborates the hospitalization picture a little more, showing the mean number of hospital admissions and the mean number of nights of inpatient care during 1982 for those hospitalized. These figures are 1.5 admissions and 10 nights, respectively.

If we multiply these figures by the 10 percent of the population hospitalized during the year, we have estimates of .15 admissions and one day per person for the population surveyed as a whole. This average number of admissions seems comparable to NCHS estimates for 1981 of .14 per person (14.2 per 100) from the 1981 social survey (NCHS, 1982 a: 25) and .16 per person (161.9 per 1000) from the 1980 hospital discharge data (NCHS, 1982 b: 97). The average number of nights in the hospital may be a little understated compared to the NCHS estimate of 1.163 days per person for 1980 (NCHS, 1982 b: 97). However, the trend from 1975 to 1980 was toward a decrease in average number of hospitalized days according to the same NCHS data, so we may expect a slightly lower number for 1982 compared to 1980.

The patterns in inpatient care are not surprising. Again, the means on both indicators seem to rise with age and possibly be higher for the poorest groups. A clear inverse relationship between average number of hospital admissions as well as average number of hospital days and income has been shown with NCHS data, although the pattern is not so evident with our somewhat smaller sample here (NCHS, 1982 b: 103).

We believe that it is important to have these baseline data and to continue to monitor these two measures (average number of hospital admissions and average number of nights in the hospital) because of current changes in the payment of hospital care by Medicare and the possibility that the same approach will be adopted by other health financial coverage plans. Briefly, the new payment plan based on diagnosis-related groups (DRGs), adopted by Medicare in January 1984, may change physician and hospital incentives in such a way as to also effect changes in the way patients are treated (see Chapter 1). The expectation, if this happens, is that patients will be hospitalized for shorter periods of time but possibly more often. The overall result may be a greater mean number of hospital days per year. It is therefore critical in this period of change to monitor three indicators: average number of hospital admissions, average length of stay and average number of hospital nights in the year. Any two of these indicators will yield the third. In this case, we present mean number of hospital admissions and mean number of nights in the hospital.

## Realized access: specific policy issues

In this section we present findings for measures of utilization of services that might be considered refinements of the measures reported above. These refinements reflect specific policy concerns. First, in light of the present concerns about cost containment, it seems appropriate to identify those groups who seem to have access according to more global indicators, but whose access is mostly to the more expensive sources of care. As in the section on the regular source of care, above, we turn our attention to outpatient department and emergency room use. Here we are concerned with actual, rather than potential, use of these sources of care. Second, in response to concerns about improving levels of health through preventive care, we will show the distribution for those who have received selected inoculations and screening tests.

Much concern has been expressed in recent years about primary care delivered in hospitals. Although hospital-based care is totally appropriate for emergencies and certain serious illnesses where specialty care is sought, cost-conscious health policymakers are striving to get ambulatory care out of the hospital (see Chapter 1). Table 2.10 gives some indication of how much ambulatory care is being received in the hospital. Column 1 shows the mean number of visits for each of the groups to the outpatient department or emergency room of a hospital during the year prior to interview; Column 2 presents, once again, the average number of visits to the doctor at all settings for the same time period, and Column 3 presents the ratio of these two (percent OPD/ER of total visits) to yield the ratio of hospital visits to the total. For the overall population, the ratio is 18. The figure is largest for Blacks (27%), the poor, especially the nonwhite poor (28%), the uninsured (26%) and the unemployed (25%).

We now turn to the issue of preventive care. In recent years policymakers have devoted much attention to this issue (e.g., Green, et al., 1983; Office of the Assistant Secretary for Health, 1979). For the measures of use reported above, we were not able to present any "expert" norms for appropriate levels, but have, rather, relied on the population average as the norm. For the measures reported here we will turn to norms published by specialists in the field.

Table 2.11 presents data for adult respondents on three indicators: the percent who had a blood pressure check in the year prior to interview, the percent of females who had a Pap smear in that year, and the percent of females who had a breast exam from a doctor. Normative data are from two sources: the American Cancer Society (1980) and the Canadian Task Force on the Periodic Health Examination (1979). These norms can be used only indirectly; that is, they are age-specific recommendations for the time intervals at which each member of the group should receive the tests. If the standards recommend every five years, for example, and the population distributes itself evenly over the year, it is appropriate to find that no more than 20 percent received the test in any given year. However, we cannot be sure that a different 20 percent will receive the test in each of the other four years. Nonetheless, these norms are an indirect way of viewing the appropriateness of public access to these preventive procedures.

The Canadian norms recommend that people receive a blood pressure check at least every five years until the age of 64, but more often if they have the opportunity (i.e., visit the doctor's office for some other reason). At age 65 this should be increased to at least every two years. Given this norm, it appears that our population is doing well, and may be receiving more blood pressure checks than necessary. The percent who receive this test increases appropriately with age. It is highest for SMSA dwellers and lowest for rural farm residents. It also increases with income. There is not a great difference between the percent of poor and nonpoor Whites who had their blood pressure checked during the year. There is a greater difference between the poor and nonpoor nonwhites, but this difference, with the poor nonwhites more apt to report a blood pressure check, is not significant (at P LE .05). The nonwhite group is, of course, predominantly Black; it would seem appropriate for Blacks to have these tests more often than Whites because they run a higher risk of hypertension. The group overall least apt to have their blood pressure checked is the uninsured.

Both the American Cancer Society and the Canadian Task Force recommend a Pap smear two years in a row for young women as soon as they become sexually active, and then, if the tests are normal, once every three years. The Canadians drop this to once every five years beginning at age 35. Were the three-year rule observed, and the population distributing itself evenly over time, 33 percent would seem to be an appropriate percentage for this test in any given year. It appears, then, that most age groups are receiving a Pap smear at levels that are not too low; the average is 60 percent. Again, one could argue, given the norms, that the levels are too high. However, it must be remembered that the percentage does not tell us whether those who did not receive the test this year will in the next two years. The likelihood of receiving a Pap smear decreases with age, with 43 percent of the oldest women receiving it. The same relationship is observed for residence and income as reported for blood pressure checks; that is, women who live in SMSAs are more apt to have a Pap smear test than women living in rural areas, and high-income women are substantially more likely to receive a Pap smear test than low-income women. The nonwhite group is more likely to receive a Pap smear than the White group. Those without insurance are somewhat less likely than average to receive a Pap smear. Those with private insurance are somewhat more likely to have a Pap smear than those insured under public programs, possibly because public programs do not necessarily cover this procedure (unless it can be linked to a diagnosis, for Medicare).

The final measure on which data were collected for adults is a physician-administered breast exam for females in the past year. The Canadian norms recommend a breast exam from a professional every year; the American Cancer Society recommends one every three years until age 40 and every year thereafter. According to the 1982 access study data, 65 percent of the women received a breast exam in that year. In addition, the percent decreased with age. We again see the pattern of rural people less likely to have this test than those living in SMSAs. We also see the familiar relationship with income which we saw for the other tests; that is, the lower the income, the less likely is the woman to receive a breast exam. People with private insurance are somewhat more likely than average to have this test, probably for the same reasons pointed out above, and people with no insurance are somewhat less likely to have it. Blacks again are at least as likely to receive this screening test as are the majority Whites.

We now turn to the preventive care delivered to children. Table 2.12 presents the percent of each group who have ever received a TB skin test, measles immunization, DPT immunization and polio immunization. The norms we used are, again, those developed by the Canadian Task Force on the Periodic Health Examination (1979) as well as those developed by the American Academy of Pediatrics (1983). The Canadian norms recommend measles, DPT and polio vaccines be given before a child reaches one year, although they always carefully specify that these inoculations should be given only to children in good health. However, the number of children left out because of poor health would presumably be no more than one or two percent. The Canadian norms repeat the requirement for initiating these series of inoculations into the early years, presumably for those children who have not yet completed the series or were not in good health earlier. The American Academy of Pediatrics would give DPT and polio vaccines during infancy, but wait until the child reached one year to give measles vaccines. The American Pediatric Association recommends the TB test be given at one year also, but here the Canadian norms diverge quite strongly to suggest it be given only if the child lives in a community where TB is likely.

The data suggest that children are not so quick to receive the measles, DPT and polio vaccines as the norms suggest, with 49 percent, 69 percent and 77 percent of the infants having received each one, respectively. By age five, the percentage is in the 90th percentile for all of the inoculations. However, if we assume that the percent that should not receive these tests is no greater than two percent, then the percent who have received measles and polio shots by this age is still below the recommended standard, although the percent receiving the DPT inoculation is quite high. By age 17, probably because of school requirements, 97 percent have received the measles and 99 percent have received the other two inoculations. There are no clear differences by the other variables defining subgroups on the these measures, with all obtaining them at about the same levels. The TB test follows a little different pattern. Only 80 percent of the children ever receive this. And we see some of the same patterns we saw for adult preventive tests, with the SMSA residents more apt to have this test (although this difference is not significant at the P LE .05 level), and an inverse relationship between the probability of receiving the test and income. Seemingly large differences between the White and nonwhite nonpoor groups were not significant.

## Realized access: patient satisfaction

Patient satisfaction measures are another way of determining the extent to which access is actually achieved. Although the utilization measures may indicate that a group has achieved access, if the group expresses dissatisfaction about some aspect of the care received, this calls into question the extent to which access was indeed obtained.

The dimensions of patient satisfaction measured in the 1982 access survey were chosen based on a number of past studies. Responses to questions about patient satisfaction with medical care tend to cluster on several dimensions. There is good evidence indicating that one of these is the cost of care, particularly the patient's personal out-of-pocket cost. Convenience of care aspects (getting an appointment, not waiting too long in the doctor's office, etc.) tend to cluster on a different dimension. Of all the items commonly asked regarding convenience, waiting time in the doctor's office is by far the most criticized. Personal characteristics of the physician or other providers (courtesy, consideration and interest in the patient) is clearly another dimension. Quality of care is apt to be perceived similarly to the personal characteristics of physicians (Aday and Andersen, 1975; Fleming, 1981; Hulka, et al., 1971; Ware and Snyder, 1975). It is important to recall as well, in examining these data, that one overriding finding in studies of patient satisfaction is that all major subgroups of the population, defined by ethnicity, age, residence, region and similar variables, report generally high levels of satisfaction with care except in those instances where the measures used are devised expressly to yield a normal distribution of responses from the population (Aday, et al., 1980: Chapter 4).

Table 2.13 presents the data from the 1982 study compared to findings from the 1976 National Survey of Access for each of the dimensions of patient satisfaction which we measured. These were selected based on the findings cited above and on our perceptions of which dimensions warranted continued monitoring. Out-of-pocket cost and office waiting time are included because they are the dimensions of care most often criticized by consumers (Aday, et al., 1980: Chapter 4). Travel time is usually not so highly criticized, but one may suspect it will be a critical issue for those who live in generally underserved areas. Time with the doctor, the information received and the patient's perceptions of quality of care are all included because they are considered critical issues in assessing the quality of care received. A final measure of the overall visit is included as a summary indicator of subjectively evaluated access. Respondents were asked for an overall evaluation of their most recent medical visit. The questions were limited to those who had a visit within the year prior to interview, to minimize recall problems and also because we are interested in evaluating care received from the *current* medical care system.

The scale on which patient responses were elicited in 1982 differed from the one used in 1976, so that the levels of dissatisfaction expressed in the two studies are not comparable. In 1982 respondents were asked to report whether they were "completely satisfied," "somewhat satisfied," or "not at all satisfied." In 1976, they were asked to report whether they were "completely satisfied," "mostly satisfied," "moderately satisfied," "slightly satisfied" or "not at all satisfied." We have, however, shown the rank ordering of the items tapped for both years in Table 2.13. In the 1982 study the groups "somewhat satisfied" and "not at all satisfied" were combined to create the percentages reported of those "not completely satisfied," whereas in 1976 the groups "moderately satisfied," "slightly satisfied" and "not at all satisfied" were combined to create the group "somewhat critical" of the medical system.

It is clear from Table 2.13 that the dimensions of care rank similarly for the two years. Out-of-pocket cost of care is still the most criticized dimension, followed by office waiting time. Information from the doctor was a less sensitive issue than time with the doctor and travel time in 1982, whereas it was the item with the third highest level of dissatisfaction in 1976. The differences in levels of criticism on these three items are not great but are significant, and could indicate a growing awareness on the part of physicians and health providers of patients' desires for complete information on their illness. The rank order on dissatisfaction of the summary measure, the overall visit, seems to have risen in 1982.

Table 2.14 shows the breakdown on dissatisfaction for 1982 by the population groups we have been examining. We do not include data from the 1976 study of access in Table 2.14 because of the difference in scale used for the responses in the two years. It is clear from Table 2.14 that, except for the youngest groups (infants, ages 1–5 and 6–17), whose responses were provided by their parents or other responsible adults, the percent not completely satisfied decreases with age on every item. This pattern is familiar, as it has been found in patient evaluations in prior years as well. There is also a consistent pattern by income, with the lowest income groups least satisfied (although differences are small). This has also been found in previous studies. Similarly, Blacks are slightly more critical than Whites on every item, also a stable finding (Aday, et al., 1980; Aday and Andersen, 1975).

Those living on farms are generally less apt to be dissatisfied than those in other residential settings. It is curious that this also appears to be the case for travel time, whereas our assumption might be that these are the people who find it difficult to obtain care within a convenient distance, and that this would affect their evaluation of travel time. Others living in rural areas seem to be relatively critical on this dimension. Those who are unemployed are consistently more critical, on each dimension, of the care received during the year. However, the group that stands out as the most critical of all, on practically every dimension, is the uninsured.

## Summary: the picture of access in 1982

In the preceding paragraphs we have presented a profile of access to medical care in the United States in 1982.

Much of the picture is similar to what we have seen before, especially in 1976, when the last national survey expressly to measure access was carried out (Aday, et al., 1980). Here we will review and discuss those findings which show change as well as those which focus on relationships not emphasized previously in studies of access to medical care.

Our exploration of potential access indicators revealed that the percent of people who have a usual source of care but not a particular doctor had increased slightly for most groups. We may only speculate as to why this happened. It could be due to the growing movement to enroll people in Health Maintenance Organizations (HMOs), where people may be less apt to see the same doctor over time. It may also be a result of the emergence of freestanding urgent care or outpatient surgery centers, in which physicians are more likely to rotate for care.

A more important question is, does it matter? We cited above a literature that pointed out that having a single doctor had the benefits of continuity which may be related to quality of care. One recent study questions this relationship (Roos, et al., 1980), and if the change in regular source of care is indeed due to more HMO-type sources, there is reasonable evidence that the HMOs provide care of quality equivalent to or better than that from the more traditional private doctor's office (Luft, 1981). We also pointed out above that past studies of access have indicated that people with a single doctor as a regular source of care are more apt to be satisfied with all aspects of their care than are people with a regular source but no particular doctor. We were not able to tell whether there has been a change in levels of satisfaction (which are, in any case, high) because of the lack of comparability between the scale used in this study and previous ones. However, this is something to monitor in the future.

Among the realized access measures, we found utilization patterns similar to those seen in earlier years. However, we did focus on some groups not examined in detail earlier. We found a particularly high average number of doctor visits for those who were covered by publicly funded programs, Medicare and Medicaid. This was not entirely an "age effect," due to the higher utilization among Medicare eligibles. Does this reflect, in part, a tendency for publicly-funded patients to have poorly coordinated followup care or be encouraged by their providers to make more visits because there is little financial loss to either patient or provider? Or is it a function of need? This will receive further study in the following chapter.

In our study of preventive care, which included another set of realized access measures, we discovered that there was little evidence that the population was receiving inadequate care, based on several indicators: blood pressure testing and Pap smear tests for adults, and measles, DPT and polio vaccinations for children. It is possible that certain individuals within each group are repeatedly not receiving the screening exams, but no group appeared definitely to be receiving these tests at lower than expected percentages according to physician-recommended norms. The same was not true for breast exams. The norms recommended that women receive a breast exam once a year, but the experience of all groups was lower than that. Nor was the level of TB testing for children high enough according to the set of U.S. norms. A fairly high percentage of children never received this test. Moreover, children received the other tests at slower than recommended rates, although by school age (probably because of school requirements) most had obtained measles, DPT and polio vaccinations.

Across many of the examined indicators, however, certain groups repeatedly were shown to have poorer access than others. These groups included, as we have seen in the past, the Blacks, the poor (especially poor Blacks), the unemployed and especially the uninsured. This was the case for all the potential access indicators (having a particular doctor as a regular source of care, waiting time in the doctor's office) and the measures of satisfaction. On the global measures of utilization, the Blacks, the poor and the unemployed did not seem to fare so badly in general, but the uninsured still stood out as a group that reflected particularly low rates. On the preventive measures, the Blacks and the poor did not, in general, seem to be more disadvantaged than the majority, affluent groups. However, women in publicly-funded programs were definitly less apt to receive Pap smears and breast exams, perhaps because these programs do not necessarily cover preventive care. Again, the uninsured were somewhat less apt to receive any of the screening tests and inoculations. They, as well as the unemployed, stood out as the least satisfied groups on most of the dimensions of satisfaction measured.

Who are these uninsured, who seem to be doing worse on more indicators than any other group studied here? Table 2.15 profiles the uninsured and compares them to the insured (those covered by private as well as public programs). (See Appendix C for the method of defining those with and without insurance coverage.) First of all, they represent about nine percent of the overall population. Those who are under 65 (almost all the people 65 and over are eligible for Medicare) represent 9.5 percent of the under-65 population (estimate not shown in table)—less than the comparable figure for 1976 (Aday and Andersen, 1978). They are overwhelmingly concentrated in the low-income and poor groups, both White and nonwhite, despite the existence of Medicaid programs targeted toward these groups. Older children and young adults are overrepresented among the uninsured as are

Hispanics and people in the central city. Not surprisingly, the unemployed are substantially overrepresented in this group. Chapter 3 will further explore the dynamics behind the key patterns described here, focusing particular attention on these and other groups who are disadvantaged in their access to medical care.

# TABLE 2.1 Percent of U.S. Population Who Had Each Type of Regular Source of Care: 1982(a), 1976(b), 1970(c)

| | TYPE OF REGULAR SOURCE OF CARE | | | | | | | | |
|---|---|---|---|---|---|---|---|---|---|
| | Percent With Particular Doctor | | | Percent With Place But No Particular Doctor | | | Percent With None | | |
| POPULATION SUBGROUPS | 1982 | 1976 | 1970 | 1982 | 1976 | 1970 | 1982 | 1976 | 1970 |
| **AGE** | | | | | | | | | |
| 1-5 | 84 | 82 | 84 | 12 | 12 | 10 | 4 | 5 | 6 |
| 6-17 | 79 | 81 | 83 | 14 | 10 | 9 | 7 | 10 | 8 |
| 18-34 | 69 | 69 | 78 | 14 | 11 | 9 | 17 | 20 | 13 |
| 35-54 | 77 | 78 | 81 | 12 | 9 | 6 | 11 | 13 | 13 |
| 55-64 | 82 | 87 | 83 | 12 | 7 | 5 | 7 | 7 | 12 |
| 65+ | 87 | 86 | 86 | 8 | 5 | 3 | 7 | 9 | 11 |
| **RESIDENCE** | | | | | | | | | |
| SMSA | 76 | – | – | 13 | – | – | 11 | – | – |
| Central City | 71 | 71 | 73 | 17 | 14 | 13 | 12 | 15 | 15 |
| Other | 79 | 77 | 84 | 11 | 10 | 6 | 10 | 13 | 10 |
| Non SMSA | 79 | – | – | 10 | – | – | 10 | – | – |
| Other Urban | – | 85 | 89 | – | 6 | 4 | – | 10 | 6 |
| Rural Non Farm | 79(e) | 84 | 86 | 10(e) | 6 | 6 | 11(e) | 10 | 8 |
| Farm | 81 | 88 | 85 | 12 | 5 | 3 | 7 | 7 | 12 |
| **FAMILY INCOME** | | | | | | | | | |
| Low | 74 | 75 | 71 | 14 | 11 | 13 | 12 | 14 | 16 |
| Medium | 74 | 77 | 83 | 14 | 10 | 7 | 12 | 13 | 10 |
| High | 81 | 82 | 87 | 11 | 7 | 5 | 8 | 11 | 8 |
| **ETHNICITY (d)** | | | | | | | | | |
| Hispanic | 72 | –(f) | –(f) | 17 | –(f) | –(f) | 11 | –(f) | –(f) |
| Non Hispanic | | | | | | | | | |
| White | 79 | 81 | 84 | 11 | 7 | 6 | 10 | 12 | 10 |
| Black | 67 | 62 | 64 | 20 | 23 | 21 | 14 | 15 | 16 |
| **150% POVERTY LEVEL BY RACE** | | | | | | | | | |
| Poor | 73 | – | – | 16 | – | – | 12 | – | – |
| White | 77 | – | – | 13 | – | – | 12 | – | – |
| Nonwhite | 64 | – | – | 24 | – | – | 12 | – | – |
| Non Poor | 78 | – | – | 12 | – | – | 10 | – | – |
| White | 79 | – | – | 11 | – | – | 10 | – | – |
| Nonwhite | 71 | – | – | 15 | – | – | 14 | – | – |
| **MAIN EARNER EMPLOYMENT STATUS** | | | | | | | | | |
| Employed | 77 | 79 | 84 | 12 | 9 | 7 | 11 | 12 | 9 |
| Not employed | 70 | 71 | 63 | 16 | 14 | 16 | 14 | 14 | 20 |
| Not in labor force | 80 | 80 | 76 | 11 | 10 | 11 | 8 | 10 | 14 |
| **INSURANCE COVERAGE** | | | | | | | | | |
| Private only | 78 | 81 | – | 12 | 8 | – | 10 | 11 | – |
| Public only | 75 | 73 | – | 16 | 15 | – | 10 | 13 | – |
| Public and private | 80 | 82 | – | 12 | 9 | – | 8 | 10 | – |
| No insurance | 59 | 64 | – | 18 | 12 | – | 22 | 23 | – |
| **TOTAL** | 77 | 78 | 81 | 12 | 9 | 8 | 11 | 12 | 11 |

(a) Percent table N is of U. S. population equals 99; percent NA equals 1.
(b) Percent table N is of U. S. population equals 99; percent NA equals 1.
(c) Percent table N is of U. S. population equals 99; percent NA equals 1.
(d) On this and subsequent tables the figures for Blacks for 1976 and 1970 are really for all nonwhites, although the percentage among those who are not Black is negligible.
(e) This figure includes both other urban and rural non farm in 1982.
(f) Hispanics are not identified for these years but are included in the White or Black groups below, as appropriate.

# TABLE 2.2  Percent of U.S. Population Who Had Each Location of Source of Care: 1982

| LOCATION OF SOURCE OF CARE | PERCENTAGE | |
|---|---|---|
| | People With a Regular Source (a) | People Without a Regular Source "Would Go" (b) |
| Doctor's Office or Private Clinic | 83% | 76% |
| Company or Union Clinic | 1 | 2 |
| School, Unspecified Clinic | 1 | 1 |
| Government Clinic | 4 | 6 |
| Hospital Outpatient Department | 8 | 9 |
| Hospital Emergency Room | 2 | 7 |
| HMO | 1 | 0 |
| Other | 1 | 0 |
| TOTAL (c) | 101% | 101% |

(a) Percent table N is of U. S. population equals 89; percent with no regular source or NA equals 11.

(b) Percent table N is of U. S. population equals 7; percent with regular source, no "would go" source, or NA equals 93.

(c) The percentages did not sum to 100 because of rounding error.

**TABLE 2.3  Percent of U.S. Population with Hospital Outpatient Department or Emergency Room as Regular Source of Care: 1982**

| POPULATION SUBGROUPS | PERCENT WITH REGULAR SOURCE AS OPD OR ER (a) |
|---|---|
| AGE | |
| 1-5 | 8 |
| 6-17 | 10 |
| 18-34 | 10 |
| 35-54 | 9 |
| 55-64 | 10 |
| 65+ | 14 |
| RESIDENCE | |
| SMSA | |
| Central City | 10 |
| Other | 14 |
| Non SMSA | 7 |
| Non Farm | 10 |
| Farm | 14 |
| FAMILY INCOME | |
| Low | 14 |
| Medium | 10 |
| High | 7 |
| ETHNICITY | |
| Hispanic | 12 |
| Non Hispanic | |
| White | 8 |
| Black | 20 |
| 150% POVERTY LEVEL | |
| BY RACE | |
| Poor | 15 |
| White | 12 |
| Nonwhite | 27 |
| Non Poor | 8 |
| White | 8 |
| Nonwhite | 14 |
| MAIN EARNER | |
| EMPLOYMENT STATUS | |
| Employed | 9 |
| Not employed | 16 |
| Not in labor force | 14 |
| INSURANCE COVERAGE | |
| Private only | 8 |
| Public only | 21 |
| Public and private | 16 |
| No insurance | 18 |
| TOTAL | 10 |

(a) Percent table N is of U.S. population equals 89; percent with no regular source or NA equals 11.

**TABLE 2.4 Percent of U.S. Adults with Different Levels of Office Waiting Time on Recent Medical Visit: 1982**

| POPULATION SUBGROUPS | OFFICE WAITING TIME ON RECENT MEDICAL VISIT (a) | | |
|---|---|---|---|
| | Percent Up To 30 Mins. | Percent Over 30 Up To 60 Mins. | Percent More Than 60 Mins. |
| AGE | | | |
| 18-34 | 82 | 12 | 6 |
| 35-54 | 84 | 11 | 5 |
| 55-64 | 80 | 14 | 6 |
| 65+ | 87 | 9 | 4 |
| RESIDENCE | | | |
| SMSA | | | |
| Central City | 84 | 11 | 5 |
| Other | 81 | 13 | 6 |
| Non SMSA | 85 | 10 | 5 |
| Non Farm | 81 | 13 | 6 |
| Farm | 86 | 12 | 2 |
| FAMILY INCOME | | | |
| Low | 79 | 14 | 7 |
| Medium | 84 | 12 | 5 |
| High | 86 | 9 | 4 |
| ETHNICITY | | | |
| Hispanic | 71 | 19 | 10 |
| Non Hispanic | | | |
| White | 85 | 11 | 4 |
| Black | 77 | 14 | 9 |
| 150% POVERTY LEVEL | | | |
| BY RACE | | | |
| Poor | 76 | 15 | 8 |
| White | 78 | 15 | 7 |
| Nonwhite | 72 | 16 | 12 |
| Non Poor | 85 | 11 | 4 |
| White | 85 | 10 | 4 |
| Nonwhite | 80 | 12 | 7 |
| MAIN EARNER | | | |
| EMPLOYMENT STATUS | | | |
| Employed | 84 | 11 | 5 |
| Not employed | 77 | 15 | 9 |
| Not in labor force | 83 | 12 | 5 |
| INSURANCE COVERAGE | | | |
| Private only | 84 | 11 | 5 |
| Public only | 84 | 9 | 7 |
| Public and private | 85 | 12 | 3 |
| No insurance | 74 | 18 | 8 |
| TOTAL | 83 | 12 | 5 |

(a) Percent table N is of U.S. adults equals 73: percent who did not report on recent visit or NA equals 27.

PERCENT WHO SAW A PHYSICIAN IN THE YEAR

| POPULATION SUBGROUPS | 1982 (a)(b) | 1976 (c) | 1970 (d) | 1963 | 1958 |
|---|---|---|---|---|---|
| **AGE** | | | | | |
| 1-5 | 92 | 87 | 75 | 75 | 73 |
| 6-17 | 77 | 69 | 62 | 58 | 64 |
| 18-34 | 83 | 77 | 70 | 67 | 68 |
| 35-54 | 76 | 75 | 67 | 65 | 64 |
| 55-64 | 81 | 79 | 73 | 68 | 66 |
| 65+ | 87 | 79 | 76 | 68 | 68 |
| **RESIDENCE** | | | | | |
|   SMSA | | | | | |
|     Central City | 83 | — | — | — | — |
|     Other | 82 | 77 | 65 | 66(g) | — |
|   Non SMSA | 78 | 78 | 72 | — | — |
|     Other urban | — | 73 | 71 | — | — |
|     Rural Non Farm | 79(e) | 75 | 68 | 66 | — |
|     Farm | 71 | 68 | 62 | 67 | — |
| **FAMILY INCOME** | | | | | |
|   Low | 80 | 73 | 65 | 56 | — |
|   Medium | 80 | 75 | 67 | 64 | — |
|   High | 84 | 79 | 71 | 71 | — |
| **ETHNICITY** | | | | | |
|   Hispanic | 80 | —(f) | —(f) | — | — |
|   Non Hispanic | | | | | |
|     White | 82 | 76 | 70 | — | — |
|     Black | 82 | 74 | 59 | — | — |
| **150% POVERTY LEVEL** | | | | | |
|   BY RACE | | | | | |
|     Poor | | | | | |
|       White | 79 | — | — | | |
|       Nonwhite | 79 | — | — | | |
|     Non Poor | | | | | |
|       White | 80 | — | — | | |
|       Nonwhite | 82 | — | — | | |
| **MAIN EARNER EMPLOYMENT STATUS** | | | | | |
|   Employed | 81 | 76 | 69 | — | — |
|   Not employed | 80 | 73 | 65 | — | — |
|   Not in labor force | 85 | 77 | 68 | — | — |
| **INSURANCE COVERAGE** | | | | | |
|   Private only | 82 | 76 | — | — | — |
|   Public only | 85 | 79 | — | — | — |
|   Public and private | 87 | 82 | — | — | — |
|   No insurance | 67 | 64 | — | — | — |
| **TOTAL** | 81 | 76 | 68 | 65 | 66 |

(a) See Appendix C for a discussion of how the physician visit question asked in 1982 differed from previous studies.
(b) Percent table N is of U.S. population equals 100; percent NA equals 0.
(c) Percent table N is of U.S. population equals 99; percent NA equals 1.
(d) Percent table N is of U.S. population equals 98; percent NA equals 2.
(e) This figure includes both other urban and rural nonfarm in 1982.
(f) Hispanics are not identified for these years and are included in the White or Black groups below, as appropriate.
(g) This figure includes central city SMSA, other SMSA and other urban non-SMSA for this year.

**TABLE 2.6 Mean Number of Physician Visits per Person Who Saw a Physician in the Year: 1982, 1976**

MEAN NUMBER OF PHYSICIAN VISITS PER PERSON WHO SAW A PHYSICIAN

| POPULATION SUBGROUPS | 1982 (a)(c) | 1976 (b)(c) |
|---|---|---|
| AGE | | |
| 1-5 | 5.7 (0.43) | 5.3 (0.27) |
| 6-17 | 4.9 (0.32) | 3.4 (0.20) |
| 18-34 | 6.2 (0.40) | 5.5 (0.24) |
| 35-54 | 6.5 (0.52) | 5.8 (0.32) |
| 55-64 | 6.9 (0.68) | 6.2 (0.43) |
| 65+ | 6.6 (0.37) | 7.6 (0.34) |
| RESIDENCE | | |
| SMSA | | |
| Central City | 6.2 (0.23) | 6.0 (0.23) |
| Other | 6.4 (0.23) | 5.3 (0.18) |
| Non SMSA | | |
| Other urban | 5.9 (0.28) | 5.4 (0.28) |
| Rural Non Farm | 6.0(d) (0.37) | 5.1 (0.27) |
| Farm | 5.5 (0.67) | 4.0 (0.29) |
| FAMILY INCOME | | |
| Low | 6.9 (0.36) | 6.3 (0.21) |
| Medium | 6.0 (0.40) | 5.3 (0.18) |
| High | 5.5 (0.35) | 4.8 (0.19) |
| ETHNICITY | | |
| Hispanic | 6.7 (0.72) | -(e) |
| Non Hispanic | | |
| White | 5.9 (0.20) | 5.3 (0.12) |
| Black | 6.7 (0.59) | 5.6 (0.37) |
| 150% POVERTY LEVEL | | |
| BY RACE | | |
| Poor | 7.5 (0.44) | -- |
| White | 7.4 (0.41) | -- |
| Nonwhite | 7.6 (1.03) | -- |
| Non Poor | 5.7 (0.11) | -- |
| White | 5.6 (0.22) | -- |
| Nonwhite | 6.3 (0.89) | -- |
| MAIN EARNER | | |
| EMPLOYMENT STATUS | | |
| Employed | 5.7 (0.21) | 4.8 (0.15) |
| Not employed | 6.4 (0.88) | 6.0 (0.59) |
| Not in labor force | 7.5 (0.46) | 7.7 (0.44) |
| INSURANCE COVERAGE | | |
| Private only | 5.6 (0.21) | 4.8 (0.15) |
| Public only | 9.9 (1.21) | 7.4 (0.52) |
| Public and private | 7.1 (0.65) | 7.8 (0.65) |
| No insurance | 6.6 (0.74) | 5.2 (0.57) |
| TOTAL | 6.1 (0.19) | 5.4 (0.11) |

(a) Percent table N is of U.S. population equals 82; percent no doctor visits or NA equals 18.
(b) Percent table N is of U.S. population equals 76; percent no doctor visits or NA equals 24.
(c) Standard errors are reported in parentheses by the respective estimates.
(d) This figure includes both other urban and rural non farm in 1982

**TABLE 2.7  Comparison of 1980 NCHS Data and 1982 Access Study Data on Percent of U.S. Population with Each Number of Doctor Visits (a)**

| POPULATION SUBGROUPS | NCHS: TOTAL POPULATION (THOUSANDS) | PERCENT WITH NUMBERS OF VISITS | | | | | | | | | |
| --- | --- | --- | --- | --- | --- | --- | --- | --- | --- | --- | --- |
| | | NONE | | 1 | | 2-4 | | 5-12 | | 13 OR MORE | |
| | | 1980 NCHS | 1982 ACCESS | 1980 NCHS | 1982 ACCESS | 1980 NCHS | 1982 ACCESS | 1980 NCHS | 1982 ACCESS | 1980 NCHS | 1982 ACCESS |
| SEX | | | | | | | | | | | |
| Male | 105,145 | 30.06% | 22.4% | 23.32% | 18.7% | 28.67% | 31.8% | 13.28% | 20.2% | 3.37% | 6.9% |
| Female | 112,778 | 20.46 | 15.0 | 21.95 | 18.3 | 31.75 | 31.6 | 19.15 | 25.3 | 5.48 | 9.9 |
| AGE | | | | | | | | | | | |
| Under 5 years | 16,036 | 9.52 | 6.1 | 16.88 | 12.0 | 40.28 | 40.2 | 27.21 | 35.0 | 4.26 | 6.6 |
| 5-14 years | 33,856 | 27.86 | 22.1 | 30.04 | 21.1 | 28.91 | 33.2 | 9.98 | 18.3 | 2.28 | 5.4 |
| 15-24 | 40,040 | 27.55 | 17.6 | 25.03 | 17.7 | 29.02 | 36.1 | 13.32 | 20.9 | 3.88 | 7.7 |
| 25-34 | 35,249 | 24.94 | 18.4 | 22.95 | 18.2 | 29.78 | 30.8 | 16.15 | 23.0 | 5.05 | 9.5 |
| 35-44 | 25,315 | 29.02 | 23.4 | 24.50 | 20.1 | 27.70 | 27.5 | 13.58 | 19.7 | 4.07 | 9.3 |
| 45-54 | 22,554 | 28.25 | 24.5 | 21.85 | 20.4 | 29.36 | 27.4 | 14.75 | 17.3 | 4.72 | 10.5 |
| 55-64 | 20,981 | 25.08 | 19.3 | 18.73 | 19.2 | 29.92 | 28.8 | 19.07 | 23.0 | 5.97 | 10.5 |
| 65-74 | 15,225 | 22.10 | 14.1 | 13.71 | 16.4 | 31.92 | 29.9 | 24.39 | 31.5 | 6.40 | 8.1 |
| 75 years and older | 8,667 | 18.00 | 10.0 | 13.19 | 18.5 | 32.51 | 28.5 | 26.64 | 31.7 | 7.05 | 11.6 |
| RACE | | | | | | | | | | | |
| White | 187,663 | 24.81 | 18.5 | 22.75 | 18.4 | 30.41 | 32.2 | 16.50 | 22.8 | 4.41 | 8.2 |
| Black | 25,585 | 26.14 | 18.1 | 21.54 | 18.8 | 29.67 | 28.8 | 15.65 | 23.6 | 4.94 | 10.7 |
| FAMILY INCOME | | | | | | | | | | | |
| Less than $5,000 | 20,319 | 22.58 | – | 17.90 | – | 30.13 | – | 20.45 | – | 7.17 | – |
| $ 5,000-$ 9,999 (b) | 31,117 | 24.91 | 19.8 | 19.44 | 17.2 | 30.17 | 29.4 | 18.71 | 23.5 | 5.19 | 10.1 |
| $10,000-$14,999 | 32,769 | 25.54 | – | 21.73 | – | 30.45 | – | 16.82 | – | 4.46 | – |
| $15,000-$24,999 | 53,254 | 25.04 | 20.3 | 23.51 | 17.9 | 30.30 | 30.3 | 15.88 | 23.4 | 4.22 | 8.1 |
| $25,000 or more | 61,515 | 23.92 | 16.4 | 25.86 | 19.9 | 31.37 | 34.5 | 14.34 | 21.9 | 3.62 | 7.3 |

(a) NCHS figures add to 98% because about 2% were classed as "unknown".  See NCHS, 1983: 34.
(b) The percentages for this category in 1982 actually include all individuals with family incomes less than $15,000.

51

## TABLE 2.8 Percent of U.S. Population Hospitalized in the Year: 1982, 1976

| POPULATION SUBGROUPS | PERCENT HOSPITALIZED IN THE YEAR | |
|---|---|---|
| | 1982 (a) | 1976 (b) |
| **AGE** | | |
| 1-5 | 8 | 10 |
| 6-17 | 3 | 5 |
| 18-34 | 12 | 12 |
| 35-54 | 10 | 12 |
| 55-64 | 10 | 15 |
| 65+ | 18 | 20 |
| **RESIDENCE** | | |
| SMSA | | - |
| Central City | 10 | 13 |
| Other | 10 | 10 |
| Non SMSA | 9 | - |
| Other Urban | - | 13 |
| Rural Non Farm | 10 (c) | 12 |
| Farm | 10 | 8 |
| **FAMILY INCOME** | | |
| Low | 12 | 13 |
| Medium | 9 | 11 |
| High | 8 | 10 |
| **ETHNICITY** | | |
| Hispanic | 9 | - (d) |
| Non Hispanic | | |
| White | 10 | 11 |
| Black | 9 | 13 |
| **150% POVERTY LEVEL** | | |
| **BY RACE** | | |
| Poor | 12 | - |
| White | 12 | - |
| Nonwhite | 12 | - |
| Non Poor | 9 | - |
| White | 10 | - |
| Nonwhite | 5 | - |
| **MAIN EARNER EMPLOYMENT STATUS** | | |
| Employed | 8 | 10 |
| Not employed | 8 | 15 |
| Not in labor force | 18 | 18 |
| **INSURANCE COVERAGE** | | |
| Private only | 9 | 10 |
| Public only | 17 | 20 |
| Public and private | 19 | 17 |
| No insurance | 6 | 9 |
| **TOTAL** | 10 | 11 |

(a) Percent table N is of U.S. population equals 99; percent infants equals 1.
(b) Percent table N is of U.S. population equals 98; percent infants or NA equals 2.
(c) This figure includes both urban and rural non farm in 1982.
(d) This figure includes both urban and rural non farm in 1982. Hispanics are not included in the White or Black groups below, as appropriate.

# TABLE 2.9 Mean Number of Hospital Admissions and Mean Number of Hospital Nights per Person Hospitalized: 1982

MEAN NUMBER OF HOSPITAL ADMISSIONS AND NIGHTS IN THE HOSPITAL DURING YEAR FOR THOSE HOSPITALIZED (a)(b)

| POPULATION SUBGROUPS | Mean Number Admissions | Mean Nights in Hospital |
|---|---|---|
| **AGE** | | |
| 1-5 | 1.3 (0.13) | 5.9 (1.90) |
| 6-17 | 1.2 (0.10) | 9.7 (3.64) |
| 18-34 | 1.4 (0.08) | 7.0 (0.86) |
| 35-54 | 1.6 (0.16) | 10.1 (1.16) |
| 55-64 | 2.0 (0.30) | 20.3 (4.68) |
| 65+ | 1.6 (0.09) | 10.4 (6.94) |
| **RESIDENCE** | | |
| SMSA | 1.6 (0.08) | 10.2 (1.04) |
| Central City | 1.5 (0.10) | 9.2 (1.53) |
| Other Urban | 1.6 (0.11) | 10.9 (1.40) |
| Non SMSA | 1.4 (0.07) | 8.8 (0.84) |
| Non Farm | 1.2 (0.08) | 9.3 (0.95) |
| Farm | | 6.6 (0.52) |
| **FAMILY INCOME** | | |
| Low | 1.6 (0.09) | 10.8 (0.97) |
| Medium | 1.3 (0.09) | 7.5 (0.71) |
| High | 1.5 (0.17) | 10.1 (2.35) |
| **ETHNICITY** | | |
| Hispanic | 1.3 (0.20) | 6.5 (0.94) |
| Non Hispanic | | |
| White | 1.5 (0.65) | 9.8 (0.87) |
| Black | 1.8 (0.20) | 12.3 (2.66) |
| **150% POVERTY LEVEL** | | |
| **BY RACE** | | |
| Poor | 1.6 (0.09) | 10.8 (1.09) |
| White | 1.6 (0.08) | 11.0 (1.02) |
| Nonwhite | 1.7 (0.24) | 10.2 (2.51) |
| Non Poor | 1.5 (0.09) | 9.4 (1.18) |
| White | 1.5 (0.10) | 9.1 (1.23) |
| Nonwhite | 2.1 (0.53) | 15.3 (6.22) |
| **MAIN EARNER EMPLOYMENT STATUS** | | |
| Employed | 1.4 (0.08) | 9.3 (1.14) |
| Not employed | 1.4 (0.16) | 6.1 (1.16) |
| Not in labor force | 1.7 (0.11) | 11.3 (1.04) |
| **INSURANCE COVERAGE** | | |
| Private only | 1.4 (0.07) | 8.8 (1.03) |
| Public only | 1.5 (0.14) | 11.7 (1.76) |
| Public and private | 1.8 (0.18) | 13.0 (1.33) |
| No insurance | 1.8 (0.43) | 6.6 (4.36) |
| **TOTAL** | 1.5 (0.06) | 10.0 (0.78) |

(a) Percent table N is of U.S. population equals 10; percent not hospitalized, infants or NA equals 90.
(b) Standard errors are reported in parentheses by the respective estimates.

**TABLE 2.10  Ratio of Hospital Outpatient Department Visits to Total Physician Visits: 1982**

| POPULATION SUBGROUPS | RATIO OF HOSPITAL OUTPATIENT DEPARTMENT VISITS TO TOTAL PHYSICIAN VISITS DURING YEAR (a) | | |
| --- | --- | --- | --- |
| | Mean OPD/ER Visits (b) | Mean Total Physician Visits (b) | Percent OPD/ER of Total Visits |
| AGE | | | |
| Infants | 0.6 (0.20) | 4.3 (0.59) | 14 |
| 1-5 | 1.0 (0.13) | 5.7 (0.43) | 18 |
| 6-17 | 0.9 (0.13) | 4.9 (0.32) | 18 |
| 18-34 | 1.3 (0.13) | 6.2 (0.40) | 21 |
| 35-54 | 1.0 (0.13) | 6.5 (0.52) | 15 |
| 55-64 | 1.2 (0.24) | 6.9 (0.68) | 17 |
| 65+ | 1.3 (0.18) | 6.6 (0.37) | 20 |
| RESIDENCE | | | |
| SMSA | 1.1 (0.08) | 6.2 (0.23) | 18 |
| Central City | 1.3 (0.15) | 6.4 (0.38) | 20 |
| Other | 1.0 (0.09) | 6.0 (0.28) | 17 |
| Non SMSA | 1.0 (0.13) | 5.9 (0.33) | 17 |
| Non Farm | 1.1 (0.15) | 6.0 (0.37) | 18 |
| Farm | 0.8 (0.16) | 5.5 (0.67) | 14 |
| FAMILY INCOME | | | |
| Low | 1.6 (0.15) | 6.0 (0.36) | 23 |
| Medium | 0.9 (0.10) | 6.0 (0.40) | 15 |
| High | 0.8 (0.09) | 5.5 (0.35) | 14 |
| ETHNICITY | | | |
| Hispanic | 1.1 (0.17) | 6.7 (0.72) | 16 |
| Non Hispanic | | | |
| White | 1.0 (0.07) | 5.9 (0.20) | 17 |
| Black | 1.8 (0.27) | 6.7 (0.59) | 27 |
| 150% POVERTY LEVEL | | | |
| BY RACE | | | |
| Poor | 1.8 (0.17) | 7.5 (0.44) | 24 |
| White | 1.7 (0.18) | 7.4 (0.41) | 23 |
| Nonwhite | 2.1 (0.26) | 7.6 (1.03) | 28 |
| Non Poor | 0.9 (0.06) | 5.7 (0.11) | 16 |
| White | 0.8 (0.06) | 5.6 (0.22) | 14 |
| Nonwhite | 1.4 (0.44) | 6.3 (0.89) | 22 |
| MAIN EARNER | | | |
| EMPLOYMENT STATUS | | | |
| Employed | 0.9 (0.06) | 5.7 (0.21) | 16 |
| Not employed | 1.6 (0.37) | 6.4 (0.88) | 25 |
| Not in labor force | 1.8 (0.23) | 7.5 (0.46) | 24 |
| INSURANCE COVERAGE | | | |
| Private only | 0.9 (0.08) | 5.6 (0.21) | 16 |
| Public only | 2.5 (0.44) | 9.9 (1.21) | 25 |
| Public and private | 1.5 (0.21) | 7.1 (0.65) | 21 |
| No insurance | 1.7 (0.32) | 6.6 (0.74) | 26 |
| TOTAL | 1.1 (0.07) | 6.1 (0.19) | 18 |

(a) Percent table N is of U.S. population equals 82; percent no doctor visits or NA equals 18.
(b) Standard errors are reported in parentheses by the respective estimates.

# TABLE 2.11 Preventive Care for Adults in the U.S. Population: 1982

POPULATION SUBGROUPS | PREVENTIVE CARE FOR ADULTS DURING THE YEAR

| | Percent With Blood Pressure Check (a) | Percent Females With Pap Smear (b) | Percent Females With Breast Exam (b) |
|---|---|---|---|
| AGE | | | |
| 18-34 | 74 | 69 | 70 |
| 35-54 | 78 | 62 | 66 |
| 55-64 | 84 | 45 | 55 |
| 65+ | 86 | 43 | 59 |
| RESIDENCE | | | |
| SMSA | | | |
| Central City | 79 | 61 | 68 |
| Other | 79 | 63 | 69 |
| Non SMSA | 79 | 61 | 67 |
| Non Farm | 74 | 55 | 58 |
| Farm | 71 | 54 | 56 |
| FAMILY INCOME | | | |
| Low | 76 | 54 | 60 |
| Medium | 77 | 61 | 66 |
| High | 80 | 66 | 71 |
| ETHNICITY | | | |
| Hispanic | 73 | 67 | 64 |
| Non Hispanic | | | |
| White | 78 | 58 | 65 |
| Black | 77 | 64 | 68 |
| 150% POVERTY LEVEL | | | |
| BY RACE | | | |
| Poor | 75 | 53 | 58 |
| White | 76 | 52 | 58 |
| Nonwhite | 72 | 58 | 61 |
| Non Poor | 79 | 62 | 68 |
| White | 78 | 61 | 68 |
| Nonwhite | 80 | 69 | 70 |
| MAIN EARNER | | | |
| EMPLOYMENT STATUS | | | |
| Employed | 77 | 64 | 68 |
| Not employed | 73 | 59 | 60 |
| Not in labor force | 84 | 46 | 58 |
| INSURANCE COVERAGE | | | |
| Private only | 79 | 65 | 70 |
| Public only | 82 | 46 | 50 |
| Public and private | 85 | 51 | 61 |
| No insurance | 64 | 48 | 48 |
| | | | |
| TOTAL | 78 | 60 | 65 |

(a) Percent table N is of U.S. adults equals 94; percent NA equals 6.
(b) Percent table N is of U.S. adult females equals 96; percent NA equals 4.

**TABLE 2.12 Preventive Care for Children in the U.S. Population: 1982**

| POPULATION SUBGROUPS | Percent With TB Skin Test | PREVENTIVE CARE FOR CHILDREN (a) | | |
|---|---|---|---|---|
| | | Percent With Measles Immunization | Percent With DPT Immunization | Percent With Polio Immunization |
| AGE | | | | |
| Infants | 32 | 49 | 69 | 77 |
| 1-5 | 73 | 91 | 98 | 94 |
| 6-17 | 85 | 97 | 99 | 99 |
| RESIDENCE | | | | |
| SMSA | 81 | 94 | 97 | 97 |
| Central City | 80 | 93 | 96 | 96 |
| Other | 82 | 94 | 98 | 97 |
| Non SMSA | 76 | 94 | 99 | 97 |
| Non Farm | 77 | 93 | 99 | 96 |
| Farm | 71 | 97 | 100 | 99 |
| FAMILY INCOME | | | | |
| Low | 76 | 94 | 98 | 97 |
| Medium | 78 | 92 | 99 | 97 |
| High | 85 | 95 | 97 | 97 |
| ETHNICITY | | | | |
| Hispanic | 80 | 93 | 97 | 96 |
| Non Hispanic | | | | |
| White | 81 | 94 | 98 | 97 |
| Black | 71 | 92 | 96 | 98 |
| 150% POVERTY LEVEL | | | | |
| BY RACE | | | | |
| Poor | 76 | 95 | 98 | 97 |
| White | 75 | 95 | 99 | 97 |
| Nonwhite | 77 | 94 | 97 | 98 |
| Non Poor | 82 | 94 | 98 | 97 |
| White | 83 | 94 | 98 | 96 |
| Nonwhite | 74 | 92 | 97 | 98 |
| MAIN EARNER | | | | |
| EMPLOYMENT STATUS | | | | |
| Employed | 80 | 94 | 98 | 97 |
| Not employed | 80 | 89 | 98 | 96 |
| Not in labor force | 79 | 95 | 95 | 98 |
| INSURANCE COVERAGE | | | | |
| Private only | 81 | 94 | 98 | 97 |
| Public only | 76 | 95 | 99 | 95 |
| Public and private | 82 | 93 | 98 | 97 |
| No insurance | 77 | 91 | 95 | 94 |
| TOTAL | 80 | 94 | 98 | 97 |

(a) Percent table N is of U.S. children equals 95; percent NA equals 5.

**TABLE 2.13  Dissatisfaction Rankings of Aspects of Medical Visit for the U.S. Population: 1982, 1976**

RANKING OF ASPECTS OF MEDICAL VISIT FROM MOST DISSATISFYING TO LEAST FOR TOTAL POPULATION

| 1982 (Percent not completely satisfied) (a) | 1976 (Percent somewhat critical) (b) |
|---|---|
| Out-of-pocket cost (40%) | Out-of-pocket cost (37%) |
| Office waiting time (31%) | Office waiting time (28%) |
| Overall visit (22%) | Information received (18%) |
| Time with doctor (21%) | Time with doctor (16%) |
| Travel time (20%) | Quality (13%) |
| Information received (18%) | Travel time (12%) |
| Quality (18%) | Overall visit (12%) |

(a) Percent table N is of U.S. population equals 70; percent with no visit in past year or NA equals 30.
(b) Percent table N is of U.S. population equals 66; percent with no visit in past year or NA equals 34.

**TABLE 2.14 Percent of U.S. Population Not Completely Satisfied with Aspects of Recent Medical Visit: 1982**

| POPULATION SUBGROUPS | Travel Time | PERCENT NOT COMPLETELY SATISFIED WITH ASPECTS OF RECENT MEDICAL VISIT (a) | | | | | |
|---|---|---|---|---|---|---|---|
| | | Office Waiting Time | Time With Doctor | Info. Received | Out-Of-Pocket Cost | Quality | Overall Visit |
| **AGE** | | | | | | | |
| Infants | 26 | 20 | 15 | 8 | 43 | 16 | 15 |
| 1-5 | 23 | 40 | 21 | 11 | 46 | 17 | 26 |
| 6-17 | 18 | 31 | 19 | 13 | 40 | 18 | 21 |
| 18-34 | 25 | 38 | 28 | 24 | 45 | 23 | 28 |
| 35-54 | 20 | 31 | 21 | 21 | 39 | 18 | 21 |
| 55-64 | 16 | 21 | 13 | 18 | 34 | 15 | 17 |
| 65+ | 13 | 19 | 12 | 12 | 31 | 13 | 13 |
| **RESIDENCE** | | | | | | | |
| SMSA | 20 | 31 | 22 | 19 | 42 | 19 | 22 |
| Central City | 20 | 32 | 22 | 19 | 41 | 19 | 24 |
| Other | 19 | 30 | 21 | 18 | 42 | 19 | 22 |
| Non SMSA | 23 | 32 | 18 | 16 | 36 | 17 | 23 |
| Non Farm | 24 | 32 | 19 | 18 | 37 | 18 | 23 |
| Farm | 18 | 32 | 13 | 7 | 30 | 12 | 19 |
| **FAMILY INCOME** | | | | | | | |
| Low | 23 | 32 | 22 | 20 | 41 | 20 | 24 |
| Medium | 19 | 31 | 20 | 18 | 40 | 18 | 22 |
| High | 19 | 31 | 20 | 17 | 40 | 17 | 22 |
| **ETHNICITY** | | | | | | | |
| Hispanic | 29 | 37 | 29 | 25 | 38 | 24 | 28 |
| Non Hispanic | | | | | | | |
| White | 19 | 31 | 20 | 17 | 40 | 17 | 21 |
| Black | 22 | 34 | 23 | 24 | 43 | 24 | 28 |
| **150% POVERTY LEVEL** | | | | | | | |
| **BY RACE** | | | | | | | |
| Poor | 23 | 34 | 24 | 22 | 40 | 22 | 26 |
| White | 23 | 33 | 24 | 21 | 40 | 21 | 26 |
| Nonwhite | 22 | 36 | 22 | 24 | 41 | 24 | 26 |
| Non Poor | 20 | 31 | 20 | 17 | 41 | 17 | 22 |
| White | 19 | 30 | 20 | 17 | 40 | 17 | 21 |
| Nonwhite | 24 | 33 | 25 | 21 | 43 | 22 | 28 |
| **MAIN EARNER** | | | | | | | |
| **EMPLOYMENT STATUS** | | | | | | | |
| Employed | 21 | 33 | 22 | 18 | 41 | 18 | 23 |
| Not employed | 26 | 38 | 28 | 22 | 46 | 28 | 30 |
| Not in labor force | 16 | 23 | 16 | 16 | 36 | 16 | 18 |
| **INSURANCE COVERAGE** | | | | | | | |
| Private only | 20 | 32 | 21 | 18 | 42 | 18 | 23 |
| Public only | 21 | 28 | 21 | 16 | 26 | 19 | 21 |
| Public and private | 16 | 27 | 15 | 16 | 34 | 17 | 19 |
| No insurance | 24 | 36 | 27 | 27 | 46 | 25 | 32 |
| **TOTAL** | 20 | 31 | 21 | 18 | 40 | 18 | 22 |

(a) Percent table N is of U.S. population equals 71; percent who did not report on recent visit or NA equals 29.

**TABLE 2.15  Profile of the Insured and Uninsured in the U.S. Population: 1982 (a)**

PROFILE OF THE INSURED AND UNINSURED (b)

| POPULATION SUBGROUPS | Percent Of Uninsured In Group | Percent of Insured In Group | Total U.S. Population |
|---|---|---|---|
| AGE | 1% | 1% | 1% |
| Infants | 1 | 1 | 1 |
| 1-5 | 8 | 8 | 8 |
| 6-17 | 23 | 18 | 19 |
| 18-34 | 35 | 30 | 30 |
| 35-54 | 17 | 23 | 22 |
| 55-64 | 14 | 10 | 11 |
| 65+ | 2 | 11 | 10 |
| RESIDENCE | | | |
| SMSA | 72 | 76 | 76 |
| Central City | 35 | 28 | 28 |
| Other | 37 | 48 | 47 |
| Non SMSA | 28 | 24 | 24 |
| Non Farm | 22 | 20 | 20 |
| Farm | 6 | 4 | 4 |
| FAMILY INCOME | | | |
| Low | 63 | 31 | 34 |
| Medium | 20 | 25 | 25 |
| High | 17 | 44 | 41 |
| ETHNICITY | | | |
| Hispanic | 16 | 8 | 8 |
| Non Hispanic | | | |
| White | 69 | 81 | 80 |
| Black | 13 | 10 | 10 |
| 150% POVERTY LEVEL | | | |
| BY RACE | | | |
| Poor | 57 | 20 | 24 |
| White | 45 | 15 | 18 |
| Nonwhite | 12 | 5 | 6 |
| Non Poor | 43 | 80 | 76 |
| White | 37 | 72 | 69 |
| Nonwhite | 6 | 7 | 7 |
| MAIN EARNER | | | |
| EMPLOYMENT STATUS | | | |
| Employed | 68 | 81 | 80 |
| Not employed | 16 | 4 | 5 |
| Not in labor force | 16 | 15 | 15 |
| TOTAL | 100 (9% of total population) | 100 (91% of total population) | 100 (100% of total population) |

(a) See Appendix C for definition of the insured and uninsured.
(b) Percents for categories within major variables (e.g., AGE, RESIDENCE, etc.) sum to 100, except for rounding error.

# Chapter 3

## Equity of Access and Its Potential for Improvement

Chapter 2 has provided both cross-sectional and trend data on major indicators of both potential and realized indicators of access to medical care. An implicit judgment in the cross-sectional comparisons between subgroups on these indicators is that the respective groups should have similar performance on the different measures. An implicit norm in the trend data comparisons is that, when controlled for need, the scores for the different groups should converge with the advent of the specific programs to improve access over time.

As indicated in the Chapter 1 discussion of the access framework to be applied in these analyses, the model can actually be used to develop a variety of standards for assessing whether access is equitable and/or appropriate as a whole or for certain target groups. In particular, there is an effort to determine whether any observed differences between certain groups are a function of differences in their respective need for care (equitable) or due to inequitable factors that can be reasonably altered by health policy (mutable) or not (immutable). Implicit judgments of what is "right" are refined and made explicit in the context of this equity of access framework.

In this chapter, this model will be tested through an examination of whether some of the key subgroup differences observed in the previous chapter are primarily a function of need or more policy-relevant inequitable factors. (A variety of other applications of the framework for measuring equity are discussed in Aday and Andersen, 1981.)

Multiple Classification Analysis (MCA), and the associated Analysis of Variance (ANOVA) and Analysis of Covariance (ANCOVA) procedures, will be used to adjust these between group differences for age, sex and need factors correlated with the access indicator of interest. (NOTE: Age and sex adjustments are included for all variables. Health status and need variables associated with the dependent (access) variable with a zero-order correlation of .05 or higher are also included.) Target group differences, based on place of residence, race, income or employment status will, in particular, be emphasized. These identify subgroups which have traditionally been disadvantaged in terms of certain access outcomes (e.g., inner city residents, the poor and racial minorities), as well as those who are apt to be particularly affected by the economic conditions of the 1970s and 1980s (e.g., the unemployed). Indicators relating to the financing (insurance coverage status) and organization (characteristics of one's regular source of care) will be considered in combination with these other factors to explore the extent to which policy changes in these areas could ultimately serve to reduce inequities observed for the respective residence, race, income and/or employment status subgroups. For the most part, the subgroup indicators represent immutable factors, though income has also been considered manipulable in some health policy indicators directed toward redistributing income.

In the tables that follow, multivariate analyses are presented for the major traditional indicators of access for which differences for these key subgroups were determined in Chapter 2. Subgroups for which no significant differences were observed are not included in the respective models. They are indicated by dashes (- -) in the data columns in the tables. Estimates adjusted for the equitable (age, sex and need) and other inequitable factors are reported for the major subgroups for which significant differences did exist in the original unadjusted estimates (see Chapter 2). In addition to the inequitable factors reflected in the subgroup comparisons, other inequitable factors which had a zero-order correlation with the access dependent variable of .05 or greater were entered in the model. These additional variables are listed in each of the tables, when applicable.

A measure of the strength of the association of the respective subgroup breakdowns and the dependent variable, adjusting for all other equitable and inequitable factors included in the model (beta), is reported for each population (residence, ethnicity, etc.) or policy-relevant (insurance coverage or regular source of care) breakdown. An adjusted F-statistic is also reported (in parentheses) for all of the variables (equitable and inequitable) entered in the model. This F-statistic is a conservative test of the statistical significance of the amount of variance in the dependent variable explained by the respective predictors, controlling for all the other variables. The F-statistic available from the SPSS ANOVA-MCA procedure, used in generating these estimates was adjusted *down* as follows, to reflect the fact that the sample was weighted and non-random (clustered):

$$\text{Fspss} * \frac{\text{Unweighted n}}{\text{Weighted n}} * \frac{1}{\text{design effect}} = \text{F adjusted.}$$

See Appendix B for a discussion of the design effect, i.e., (design factor)$^2$, relevant for the respective dependent variables and subgroup breakdowns. In general, the most conservative factor was used; that is, one that was associated with the variable in the model that had the *highest* design effect overall. As indicated earlier, inequitable factors, besides the standardized population subgroup breakdowns and regular source and insurance coverage variables which had zero-order correlations with the access (dependent) variable of .05 or greater were also entered in the respective models. These inequitable factors and the equitable (need-related) factors included in the final model are listed in the tables as well. The adjusted F-statistic for each of these variables is noted in parentheses beside it. The adjusted Fs for all variables entered in the final model were compared with Tables of the F-statistic significant at .05. Those which are significant (P LE .05) are noted with an asterisk (*) beside the adjusted F. Comparisons of the adjusted F values of all variables entered in the final model reflect the relative importance of the individual factors in explaining the access indicator of interest, when all the other variables are controlled for. In the SPSS ANOVA-MCA procedure, betas are reported only for categoric factors, but not for continuous interval-level variables entered as covariates. Hence, the adjusted F-statistic is more informative of the comparative importance of *all* the variables (both categoric and continuous) entered in the final model. The overall (total) population estimate for the access indicator of interest is reported at the bottom of the table. The total amount of variance explained by the model is reported underneath the population estimate, to provide an idea of the extent to which the factors included in the model explain the variation observed in the access measure of interest.

The findings reported in the tables that follow are grouped according to whether they refer to the organization and convenience of care or to the utilization of and satisfaction with care.

## Potential access

Table 3.1 reflects the percent with a regular source of care; those who actually see a particular doctor; those with a regular source that is a hospital outpatient department or emergency room; and the proportion with an office waiting time of 30 minutes or less at their regular source of care.

Length of time in the community, a relatively immutable inequitable factor, is significantly associated with whether people have a regular source of care, as indicated by the adjusted F value (5.04*). This suggests that people who are new to the community may be less likely to be affiliated with a regular provider and are, therefore, very likely target groups for new providers opening in the area. None of the other equitable or inequitable factors are significantly associated with reporting a regular source of care. Age (under 6) and sex have the next highest F-values, followed by insurance coverage, which also has the strongest association (highest beta) of any of the population subgroup breakdowns. The adjusted estimates for this breakdown suggest the uninsured are least likely to have a regular source of care, compared to those with some form of coverage. Only four percent (4%) of the variance is explained by this model; a combination of other inequitable or attitudinal factors not included in the model may also help account for why people do not have a particular place to go for care.

Length of time in the community continues to be the most significant predictor of whether people see one particular provider as a regular source of care. Women are also more likely than men to see a particular physician. None of the other factors are significantly associated, though age (under 6) has the next highest F value, followed by insurance coverage, which also has the strongest beta (.12) of the major subgroups considered. The uninsured tend to be much less likely to have an identifiable provider than the privately insured in particular, controlling for a variety of other factors. Around seven percent of the variance in this indicator is accounted for by the variables considered here.

Perceived health has the highest adjusted F of any variables considered in the model to explain who uses a hospital outpatient department or emergency room as a regular source of care, though none is significantly associated. The insurance coverage and race by poverty level breakdowns have the next highest F values. These variables also have the strongest associations (highest betas) of any of the breakdowns considered. The privately insured are least likely to use hospital outpatient departments or emergency rooms as a regular source of care, whereas almost a fourth (23%) of the minority poor do so. Given the judgment that such a location is not an appropriate primary source of routine medical care, it appears that poor minorities continue to be disadvantaged along this access dimension. Five percent of the variance is explained by this model.

Ethnicity has the strongest association with the length of time spent waiting to see a physician during the patient's most recent medical visit. Hispanics are much less likely to have short waits of half an hour or less than are other racial groups—particularly majority Whites. The location of one's regular source of care was the other inequitable factor with a comparable strength of association (beta). Hospital outpatient department or emergency room users tend to have the longest waits. The findings on this indicator support the conclusion that certain minorities, especially those who use hospital outpatient departments or emergency rooms, continue to have the least convenient access. Five percent of the variance in waiting time is explained by the variables considered here.

## Realized access

Table 3.2 provides data on various indicators of the utilization of health services, adjusted for both equitable and inequitable factors.

The equitable factors are the most important predictors of whether a physician was seen in the year—age (under 6), sex and disability days. However, even adjusting for these equitable factors, significant differences continue to persist according to insurance coverage and type of regular source of care. Around two-thirds of those who did not have a regular source reported going to a physician, compared to over three-fourths or more (77% to 84%) of those with a regular source. Previous research has suggested the causal importance of having a regular source of care in predicting utilization of health services (Andersen and Aday, 1978). After other equitable and inequitable factors are adjusted for, the uninsured were still less likely to have contacted a doctor in the past year. For this important indicator of realized access, it appears that organizational and financing factors do make a difference. There is evidence, then, that some inequities do continue to exist along this important access dimension, though traditional racial and income differentials *per se* are of less importance than was the case in previous years. Eight percent of the variance in this indicator is explained by the factors considered here.

Equitable factors—particularly need, as reflected in perceived health and the number of disability days reported in the year—continue to be the strongest predictors of the overall number of visits, once people are seen by a physician. None of the inequitable factors are significantly associated, though the association of insurance coverage status with the volume of visits estimate is the strongest of the ones considered. Even after adjustments for equitable and other inequitable factors, the average number of visits for individuals who only have public coverage remains high. This may reflect the tendency of physicians to encourage publicly-insured patients—most of whom are covered for outpatient ambulatory care—to return for followup care more often than people with private insurance (who are less likely to be covered for outpatient physician services) or those with no coverage at all. Or, on the contrary, it may reflect a profile of care for public aid or Medicare patients of doctor shopping or discontinuous or poorly coordinated followup care. The findings here signal the important concerns about high utilization rates for this group, but the most appropriate explanation cannot be determined on the basis of the data available in this study. Around eight percent of the variation in physician use rates is explained by the factors considered in this model.

Whether a person is hospitalized in the year appears to be primarily a function of equitable factors, as reflected in the significant impact of the number of disability days and perceived health on this indicator. None of the inequitable factors are significantly associated. For this indicator then services are relatively equitably distributed. Nine percent of the variance is explained by this model.

Disability days are significantly associated with whether or not adults had a blood pressure check in the year. The most important inequitable predictor was whether the person had a regular source of care. People with no regular source were much less likely to have had a blood pressure check than those with a regular family doctor. Six percent of the variance is explained here.

In summary, variance in utilization rates is quite often accounted for by equitable (need-related) factors. Race and income differentials are less significant than was true in past years. However, the form of insurance coverage and type of place to which one usually goes for care continue to have substantial impact on selected outpatient physician contact rates in particular.

Table 3.3 summarizes the percent who were not completely satisfied with aspects of the most recent medical visit, including the waiting time in the doctor's office, the out-of-pocket cost to them and the overall quality of care they felt they received during the visit.

Age (over 64) was, to some extent, a significant predictor of satisfaction with office waiting time. The elderly tend to be the most satisfied. Of the inequitable factors examined to explain satisfaction with this dimension of care, the actual office waiting time was clearly the most important predictor. Twenty percent of the variance was explained by this model.

The location of one's regular source of care is the strongest predictor of satisfaction with out-of-pocket cost. Dissatisfaction is lowest for patients who go to places other than the doctor's office or hospital outpatient department or emergency room for care—e.g., a company or school clinic or government or neighborhood-sponsored facility. In these types of locations, the actual out-of-pocket cost of care is apt to be less as well. (The actual out-of-pocket cost is not available in this study.) Only three percent of the variance is explained by the factors considered here. It could be expected to be much higher if the actual cost information were available as well.

Dissatisfaction with quality is significantly associated with perceived health and length of time in the community. Dissatisfaction is lowest for people who have the best health and who are relative newcomers to the area. There do not appear to be significant differences by any of the other subgroups, though there is a tendency for people who see a particular doctor at their regular source of care to be least dissatisfied. Only four percent of the variation in satisfaction with quality is explained by these indicators.

## Summary: the profile of equity

The preceding analyses examine the extent to which differences for key population subgroups on major access performance indicators are a function of equitable or inequitable factors. To the extent need-related factors account for most of the differences observed, equity is said to exist. Differences attributable to inequitable factors may be either mutable (manipulable by health policy) or immutable (not easily changed). The mutable characteristics include both the organization and financing dimensions of care, expressed here in terms of characteristics of respondents' regular source of care or insurance coverage, respectively. These are factors which health policy initiatives could conceivably alter to some extent to try to improve access. The inequitable factors (residence, race and poverty level or employment status, for example), are not readily changed by health policy. Nonetheless, they can be used to identify the groups to whom programs might be most meaningfully applied.

Table 3.4 attempts to summarize the results of these equity-of-access analyses. (See the footnote in Table 3.4

for the critieria used in this summary.) It is apparent that for many of the indicators some of the differences observed for key target groups are a function of equitable, need-related factors. This is particularly the case for the utilization and satisfaction indicators. Some subgroup differences on these measures were diminished when need-related factors were entered as controls.

Residence, ethnicity, poverty level by race and employment status have little or no impact on most indicators when other factors are controlled for. Hispanics do, however, average longer office waiting times than do other races, especially majority whites. The differences by residence and poverty level by race are not statistically significant. Some of the traditional subgroup differences in equity, then, appear to be less salient in 1982, when relevant other (equitable and inequitable) factors are controlled for.

However, insurance coverage and whether one has a regular source and, if so, where they might go continue to be important correlates of many of the key access outcomes. Insurance coverage, for example, tends to relate to the kinds of places respondents usually go for care and their overall utilization of services. The uninsured tend to be most consistently disadvantaged in terms of the respective indicators.

People who routinely go to hospital outpatient departments or emergency rooms report the longest waiting times for care. Those who have no regular source tend to have lower utilization rates. Also, levels of satisfaction vary according to where people usually get their care. Those who see one particular doctor at his or her office register the least dissatisfaction with the overall quality of care. Satisfaction with the out-of-pocket costs of care is greatest for users of company or school clinics or neighborhood or government-sponsored clinics.

In summary, though it appears many of the traditional access inequities have diminished, there are still differing patterns of care depending on where one usually goes for medical care and if one has insurance.

Other special access problems encountered by these and other groups will be explored in the next chapter.

**TABLE 3.1 Potential Access: Organization and Convenience of Care, Adjusted for Equitable and Inequitable Factors: 1982**

| | POTENTIAL ACCESS: | | ORGANIZATION AND CONVENIENCE OF CARE | |
|---|---|---|---|---|
| | Percent with a Regular Source of Care | Percent with a Particular Doctor as Regular Source of Care | Percent of Those with a Regular Source That is Hospital OPD or ER | Percent with Office Waiting Time of 30 Minutes or Less |
| Equitable Factors (Adj. F) | Under 6 (3.16)<br>Over 64 (1.33)<br>Sex (3.79) | Under 6 (3.34)<br>Over 64 (1.49)<br>Sex (4.61*) | Over 64 (.06)<br>Sex (.76)<br>Perceived health (2.94)<br>Disability days (.22) | Over 64 (2.51)<br>Sex (.09)<br>Perceived health (3.48) |
| **Inequitable Factors** | | | | |
| **RESIDENCE** | | | | |
| SMSA | | | | |
| Central City | 88 | 72 | 13 | -- |
| Other | 90 | 79 | 8 | -- |
| Non SMSA | | | | |
| Non Farm | 88 | 78 | 10 | -- |
| Farm | 91 | 80 | 15 | -- |
| Beta (Adj F) | .03( .18) | .08(1.20) | .07( .89) | -- |
| **ETHNICITY** | | | | |
| Hispanic | 89 | 75 | -- | 71 |
| Other | 89 | 77 | -- | 84 |
| Beta (Adj F) | .00( .00) | .01( .11) | -- | .10(4.05*) |
| **150% POVERTY LEVEL BY RACE** | | | | |
| Poor | | | | |
| White | 89 | 77 | 10 | 79 |
| Nonwhite | 87 | 66 | 23 | 76 |
| Non Poor | | | | |
| White | 90 | 78 | 9 | 84 |
| Nonwhite | 85 | 73 | 12 | 85 |
| Beta (Adj F) | .04( .30) | .07( .94) | .11(1.72) | .07( .58) |

**TABLE 3.1 (continued) Potential Access: Organization and Convenience of Care, Adjusted for Equitable and Inequitable Factors: 1982**

| | Time in community, Family size (5.04*) (3.46) | Time in community (9.52*) | Education of main earner (.80) | Region (1.25) |
|---|---|---|---|---|
| MAIN EARNER | | | | |
| EMPLOYMENT STATUS | | | | |
| Employed | 89 | 77 | 10 | -- |
| Not employed | 87 | 75 | 11 | -- |
| Not in labor force | 91 | 79 | 10 | -- |
| Beta (Adj F) | .03( .25) | .02( .09) | .01( .01) | -- |
| INSURANCE COVERAGE | | | | |
| Private only | 90 | 79 | 8 | 83 |
| Public only | 89 | 71 | 18 | 86 |
| Public and private | 90 | 74 | 18 | 83 |
| No insurance | 78 | 63 | 17 | 78 |
| Beta (Adj F) | .11(2.16) | .12(2.28) | .14(1.73) | .04( .18) |
| REGULAR SOURCE | | | | |
| Doctor's Office. Particular MD | -- | -- | -- | 84 |
| Doctor's Office. No Particular MD | -- | -- | -- | 90 |
| Hospital OPD or ER | -- | -- | -- | 72 |
| Other Place | -- | -- | -- | 85 |
| No Regular Source | -- | -- | -- | 79 |
| Beta (Adj F) | -- | -- | -- | .11(1.24) |
| Other Inequitable Factors (Adj F) | | | | |
| TOTAL | 89% | 77% | 10% | 83% |
| $R^2$ | .04 | .06 | .05 | .05 |

**TABLE 3.2 Realized Access: Utilization of Services, Adjusted for Equitable and Inequitable Factors: 1982**

REALIZED ACCESS: UTILIZATION OF SERVICES

| | Percent Seeing a Physician in the Year | Mean Visits for Those Seeing a Physician | Percent Hospitalized in the Year | Percent of Adults with Blood Pressure Check |
|---|---|---|---|---|
| Equitable Factors (Adj F) | Under 6 (18.10*)<br>Over 64 (1.57)<br>Sex (19.39*)<br>Perceived health (3.08)<br>Disability days (11.12*) | Under 6 (.29)<br>Over 64 (2.17)<br>Sex (1.62)<br>Perceived health (13.06*)<br>Disability days (28.02*) | Under 6 (1.00)<br>Over 64 (1.64)<br>Sex (2.00)<br>Perceived health (5.93*)<br>Disability days (40.82*) | Over 64 (3.13)<br>Sex (2.98)<br>Perceived health (.94)<br>Disability days (4.82*) |
| **Inequitable Factors** | | | | |
| **RESIDENCE** | | | | |
| SMSA | | | | |
| Central City | 82 | -- | -- | -- |
| Other | 83 | -- | -- | -- |
| Non SMSA | | | | |
| Non Farm | 78 | -- | -- | -- |
| Farm | 72 | -- | -- | -- |
| Beta (Adj F) | .06(2.25) | | | |
| **ETHNICITY** | | | | |
| Hispanic | -- | -- | -- | -- |
| Other | -- | -- | -- | -- |
| Beta (Adj F) | -- | | | |
| **150% POVERTY LEVEL BY RACE** | | | | |
| Poor | | | | |
| White | -- | 6.0 | 10 | 75 |
| Nonwhite | -- | 6.2 | 8 | 70 |
| Non Poor | | | | |
| White | -- | 5.8 | 9 | 79 |
| Nonwhite | -- | 5.8 | 5 | 83 |
| Beta (Adj F) | | .01(.02) | .04(.44) | .06(.97) |

76

**TABLE 3.2 (continued) Realized Access: Utilization of Services, Adjusted for Equitable and Inequitable Factors: 1982**

| | | | | |
|---|---|---|---|---|
| **MAIN EARNER EMPLOYMENT STATUS** | | | | |
| Employed | -- | 6.0 | 9 | 77 |
| Not employed | -- | 5.6 | 7 | 77 |
| Not in labor force | -- | 5.5 | 11 | 81 |
| Beta (Adj F) | .06(9.89*) | .02(.08) | .03(.27) | .03(.30) |
| **INSURANCE COVERAGE** | | | | |
| Private only | 82 | 5.5 | 9 | 79 |
| Public only | 83 | 9.5 | 11 | 77 |
| Public and private | 84 | 7.3 | 13 | 79 |
| No insurance | 69 | 6.0 | 6 | 68 |
| Beta (Adj F) | .06(4.53*) | .10(1.42) | .05(.62) | .07(1.54) |
| **REGULAR SOURCE** | | | | |
| Doctor's Office, Particular MD | 84 | 6.0 | 10 | 82 |
| Doctor's Office, No Particular MD | 77 | 5.9 | 6 | 76 |
| Hospital OPD or ER | 81 | 5.8 | 10 | 77 |
| Other Place | 84 | 6.2 | 9 | 77 |
| No Regular Source | 65 | 4.9 | 6 | 59 |
| Beta (Adj F) | .15(9.89*) | .03(.19) | .05(.58) | .18(7.69*) |
| **Other Inequitable Factors (Adj F)** | Education of main earner (1.33) | | Education of main earner (.58) | |
| **TOTAL** | 81% | 6.1 | 10% | 78% |
| $R^2$ | .08 | .08 | .09 | .06 |

**TABLE 3.3  Realized Access: Satisfaction with Recent Medical Visit, Adjusted for Equitable and Inequitable Factors: 1982**

| Equitable Factors (Adj F) | Percent Not Completely Satisfied With Office Waiting Time | Percent Not Completely Satisfied With Out-of-Pocket-Cost | Percent Not Completely Satisfied With Quality of Care |
|---|---|---|---|
| | Over 64 (11.08*) | Under 6 ( .46 ) | Over 64 ( 3.29 ) |
| | Sex ( 2.46 ) | Over 64 ( 3.55 ) | Sex .52 |
| | | Sex ( .00 ) | Perceived health (10.54*) |
| | | | Disability days ( .04 ) |
| **Inequitable Factors** | | | |
| RESIDENCE | | | |
| SMSA | | | |
| Central City | — | 41 | — |
| Other | — | 41 | — |
| Non SMSA | | | |
| Non Farm | — | 38 | — |
| Farm | — | 29 | — |
| Beta (Adj F) | — | .05(1.03) | — |
| ETHNICITY | | | |
| Hispanic | — | — | 22 |
| Other | — | — | 18 |
| Beta (Adj F) | — | — | .03( .75) |
| 150% POVERTY LEVEL | | | |
| BY RACE | | | |
| Poor | | | |
| White | — | — | 19 |
| Nonwhite | — | — | 21 |
| Non Poor | | | |
| White | — | — | 17 |
| Nonwhite | — | — | 18 |
| Beta (Adj F) | — | — | .03( .13) |

**TABLE 3.3 (continued)  Realized Access: Satisfaction with Recent Medical Visit, Adjusted for Equitable and Inequitable Factors: 1982**

| | | | |
|---|---|---|---|
| MAIN EARNER | | | |
| EMPLOYMENT STATUS | | | |
| Employed | 32 | 39 | 18 |
| Not employed | 35 | 45 | 24 |
| Not in labor force | 27 | 41 | 17 |
| Beta (Adj F) | .04( .74) | .03( .47) | .04( .54) |
| | | | |
| INSURANCE COVERAGE | | | |
| Private only | 31 | 40 | 18 |
| Public only | 34 | 29 | 16 |
| Public and private | 32 | 38 | 20 |
| No insurance | 27 | 45 | 19 |
| Beta (Adj F) | .03( .23) | .05( .96) | .02( .11) |
| | | | |
| REGULAR SOURCE | | | |
| Doctor's Office, Particular MD | 30 | 41 | 16 |
| Doctor's Office, No Particular MD | 32 | 43 | 21 |
| Hospital OPD or ER | 38 | 35 | 26 |
| Other Place | 28 | 24 | 21 |
| No Regular Source | 35 | 46 | 25 |
| Beta (Adj F) | .06(1.03) | .09(2.46*) | .10(1.54) |
| | | | |
| Other Inequitable Factors (Adj F) | Time in community (1.50) | Time in community ( .75) | Time in community (6.39*) |
| | Office waiting time (108.88*) | Family size (3.31) | |
| | | | |
| TOTAL | 31% | 40% | 18% |
| $R^2$ | .20 | .03 | .04 |

**TABLE 3.4 Summary of the Impact of Equitable and Inequitable Factors on Access (a)**

| ACCESS | EQUITABLE (NEED) | INEQUITABLE | | | | MUTABLE | |
| --- | --- | --- | --- | --- | --- | --- | --- |
| | | IMMUTABLE | | | | | |
| | | Residence | Ethnicity | Poverty Level and Race | Employment Status | Insurance Coverage | Regular Source |
| Regular Source or Not | – | – | – | – | – | Yes | NA |
| Particular Doctor as Regular Source | Yes* | – | – | – | – | Yes | NA |
| Hospital OPD or ER as Regular Source | – | – | – | Yes | – | Yes | NA |
| Office Waiting Time LE 30 minutes | – | – | Yes* | – | – | – | Yes |
| Saw Doctor in Year | Yes* | – | – | – | – | Yes* | Yes* |
| Mean Doctor Visits for those with visit | Yes* | – | – | – | – | Yes | – |
| Hospitalized in Year | Yes* | – | – | – | – | – | – |
| Blood Pressure Check in Year | Yes* | – | – | – | – | – | Yes* |
| Not Completely Satisfied with | | | | | | | |
| Office Waiting Time | Yes* | – | – | – | – | – | – |
| Out-of-Pocket Cost | – | – | – | – | – | – | Yes* |
| Quality of Care | Yes* | – | – | – | – | Yes | Yes |

(a) For the equitable factors, a Yes* means at least one of the factors (age, sex or need) was significantly associated with the dependent variable. P LE .05. For the inequitable factors a Yes (without an asterisk) means the factor was associated with a beta of .09 or greater. An asterisk (yes*) indicates the adjusted F for this factor was significant. P LE .05.

# Chapter 4

## Special Access Problems in the 1980s

As mentioned in Chapter 1, the 1970s and 1980s have brought a number of economic and political changes that may well have the greatest impact on those traditionally disadvantaged groups whom we saw in previous chapters had made gains over the past 20 years but for whom some inequities continue to exist.

In this chapter special access problems encountered by U.S. families will be examined. Particular attention will be given to some of the same population subgroups for whom the major social-indicator measures of access have been analyzed to provide a fuller picture of the range of access issues of importance early in the 1980s. The indicators examined in this chapter were introduced in the 1982 access survey; comparable data from previous studies are generally not available for comparison. Therefore, we cannot make direct objective judgments, as was possible in Chapter 2 in particular, about whether access along these dimensions has improved or worsened. We can, however, show how various subgroups compare as major cost-conscious debates over health policy alternatives continue to dominate the establishment of national health care priorities. Particular emphasis will be given in the findings and discussion to the *financial* correlates and outcomes of the access problems encountered by American families during this period.

## Potential access problems

*Potential* access problems refer to those factors which *may* make it more difficult for families to obtain care, while *realized* access problems may be defined as having services reduced or finding the actual receiving of care unsatisfactory for some reason. Precise indicators of these respective concepts are not always clearly categorized as one or the other. In this chapter realized access measures will focus on the actual experience of obtaining care in response to illness, whereas the potential measures more broadly consider factors that may eventually affect the ability to obtain care.

Table 4.1 points out the proportion of U.S. families who said they found it "more difficult," compared to those who found it "easier," to obtain care this year compared to previous years. A positive score for the "Net Percent" means *more* said they found it difficult. A negative score means *fewer* found it difficult. This measure is a subjectively determined estimate of whether things have gotten better or worse in terms of a family's potential access to services.

Six percent of American families (about 4.2 million) thought it was harder to get care, while four percent (2.8 million) thought it was easier. Eleven percent of nonpoor minority families thought it was easier to obtain care, while eight percent found it more difficult to get care in

1982 than in the past. Seventeen percent of families in which the main wage earner was unemployed considered it more difficult to obtain care. A comparable proportion of families in which the random adult interviewed in the study had no insurance coverage (sixteen percent) found it more difficult to obtain care in 1982. These findings underscore the importance of family finances in predicting whether families are apt to experience more or fewer problems in getting care. The same holds true for income and poverty level. Eight percent of the low-income families said it was more difficult to obtain care—compared to four percent of those with higher incomes. When families who thought it was harder to obtain care were asked why, they most often cited financial reasons (68%), followed by convenience (26%) and other factors (5%).

Table 4.2 presents data probing somewhat more deeply into financial problems related to illness experienced by American families. About five percent of U.S. families (3.5 million) reported some loss of family earnings as a result of a family member's illness. About one-third of those reported this was a serious problem. Once again, the poor, the unemployed, those whose main wage earner was not in the labor force, or those with adults with no insurance or public coverage only experienced the most problems. In fact, in some instances, they were denied or refused care because they did not have adequate financial resources to pay for the services they needed. For example, half or more of the poor (50%), especially the minority poor (61%), those not in the labor force (54%), those who had public coverage only (67%), and those with no insurance (57%) reported that their reduced earnings resulted in serious financial problems for their family.

In Table 4.3 data are presented on the proportion of U.S. adults whose insurance coverage changed in the year. There are also data showing how the fact that coverage was dropped or reduced may have affected their ability to obtain care. About 21 percent of American adults (over 35 million) experienced changes in insurance coverage during the year—i.e., coverage was dropped, reduced or increased; the price of the policy changed, or the respondent changed companies. The percentages for whom coverage was dropped or reduced versus those with increased coverage and the net difference between the two are reported in Table 4.3. A positive score for the net difference means there were *more* for whom coverage increased. A negative score means there were proportionately *fewer* for whom there was an increase. For 39 percent coverage was increased, while for 26 percent coverage was dropped or reduced. Overall, U.S. adults who had a change in coverage experienced a positive (net) difference. Thirteen percent more had an increase than had a decrease in coverage. The variation by subgroup was, however, not always similarly positive.

Older adults (55–64 years of age) experienced less favorable shifts (−4%) than did other age groups, for whom there was more likely to be an increase in coverage. SMSA residents living outside central city areas more often experienced increased (44%) rather than diminished coverage (23%), whereas non-SMSA residents experienced fewer net changes overall (+3%). The low-income and the poor, especially poor minorities, were more apt to have their coverage dropped or reduced (52 % versus 22 % for whom it increased), while the nonpoor were more likely to increase their coverage (41% versus 24% for whom it decreased). The employed were much more likely to have experienced an increase in coverage (43%) than were those who were not employed (24%) or not in the labor force (22%). For those with jobs, the *net* increase (19%) was correspondingly much more favorable than for the unemployed ($-13\%$) or those not in the labor force ($-6\%$). The vast majority (83%) of those presently uninsured said their coverage had been dropped in the past year, demonstrating that, for many of the uninsured, the loss in benefits was recent. Those with some form of private coverage were much more apt to have improved benefits (net difference of 20%), while those with public coverage alone ($-31\%$) or no insurance at all ($-83\%$) were more likely to experience a net reduction in benefits in the year.

Twenty-three percent of those whose coverage was dropped or reduced indicated they put off care, and ten percent said they did not obtain it at all as a result of the change. The elderly were less likely than other age groups to put it off. About a third (34%) of inner city residents tended to put off getting care. Poor people were much more likely to be unable to get care (23%) than were the nonpoor (6%). The estimates for some of the ethnic groups are not very stable because of small cell sizes. There was a tendency, however, for Hispanics to put off care. Individuals in families in which the main wage earner was unemployed were much more likely to forego care (25%) than those who were employed (8%) or not in the labor force (12%). The same was true of those with no insurance (36%), particularly compared to those with some form of private insurance (4% to 6%). People who only had publicly subsidized coverage (23%) or no insurance (23%) tended to be more likely than those who had some form of private insurance (7% to 8%) to have to change the place they usually went to for care when their coverage changed, suggesting that public aid recipients, as well as those with no insurance at all, may be less able to buy their way into some settings for care than are patients who are better able to pay.

## Realized access problems

The following discussion focuses in particular on instances in which U.S. families or individuals had an illness for which they wanted or needed to seek care but encountered problems actually getting it.

For about six percent of U.S. families (4.2 million) there were times in the previous year in which someone in the family needed care but was not able to obtain it (Table 4.4). Fifteen percent of families in which the sample adult was uninsured experienced this problem, compared to five percent of the families in which the individual was privately insured. Around 40 percent of those families who needed care but did not obtain it actually tried to get care. Those least likely to try were ones in which the main wage earner was unemployed. Only one in five (20%) of these families made some effort to obtain the required service.

Table 4.5 summarizes the reasons families who said they needed care but did not obtain it cited for not going to the doctor—both those who tried and those who did not. Financial factors or the absence of insurance coverage were quite frequently cited as reasons for not going or not even trying to obtain care. Subgroup breakdowns are not provided because the cell sizes for many groups are too small to permit reliable estimates.

Five percent (3.5 million families) who had needed certain kinds of special services in the year (such as emergency medical care, overnight hospital care, a visiting nurse, mental health services, etc.) reported that they had not been able to obtain them (Table 4.6). The problems mentioned most often were finding a drug store open at night or on weekends (56%), getting a pediatrician (22%) or locating emergency care when they needed it (21%). Once again, cell sizes are too small to report subgroup breakdowns.

Families in which there was a seriously ill family member represent perhaps one of the most important groups in considering target populations in particular need of the services of the health care system. Table 4.7 shows that about nine percent of American families (over six million) had at least one seriously ill family member. One out of ten of these families had more than one seriously ill family member. Families with an ill member were more often ones in which the main wage earner was not in the labor force (16%) or with some form of public insurance (15% to 17%), reflecting the fact that such families are often headed by an elderly or disabled person.

In public aid families, in which the sampled adult was insured only through public sources, there was much more likely to be a need for additional support services in the family's home to care for the patient (43%) than was true for those with some form of private insurance (13% to 17%) or no insurance at all (17%). Major personal changes tended to be more often required in families in which the main wage earner was unemployed (24%) than in those whose head was in the work force, for example (12%). Having to stop working was often required of a family member. Asking a relative to move in to assist in the care of the seriously ill individual was necessary in many families as well.

Families were asked if they were unable to get any special services they needed to care for the person, such as a physical therapist, mental health counselor, housekeeper, etc. About 11 percent of the families with a seriously ill family member said this was a problem. Most often needed was transportation; a visiting mental health counselor or social worker; a housekeeper, or medical appliances for home use. Over a fourth (26%) of poor minorities and the publicly-insured had problems. The low-income (16%), and those families whose main wage earner was not in the labor force (17%) were more likely to have problems than were higher income families (6%). For one in five of the families (22%) a family member's illness created serious financial problems. Poor minorities were particularly affected (50%), as were Hispanics (39%) and those in which the sampled adult had no insurance coverage (52%).

Medical emergencies represent another demand on the health care system in which access barriers should be minimized as much as possible. About 15 percent of the U.S. population (34 million people) experienced such an emergency in the previous year (Table 4.8). Young children were most likely to experience these emergencies. In the overwhelming majority of the cases (77%), care was sought in a hospital outpatient department or emergency room. Only five percent of the time were there significant problems in getting to care—most often because the person needed help getting to the source of care or the traffic was slow. People seemed least satisfied with the amount of time they had to wait to see the doctor, once they were there (Table 4.9). Travel time was for the most part satisfactory, however, as was the time spent with the doctor, the quality of care and the overall visit. The uninsured tended to be most dissatisfied with most aspects of care. Hispanics and other minorities were less satisfied with the amount of time they had to wait for care, perhaps reflecting the fact that majority whites' physicians meet them at the emergency room or that minority patients may experience longer queuing than majority white patients because of overt or implicit discrimination.

## Summary: groups in trouble

The previous discussion has provided data on a variety of indicators of special access problems experienced by

U.S. families, and the earlier chapters discussed the experience of selected subgroups according to traditional measures of access. Table 4.10 summarizes results across a number of these dimensions, reflecting the families who may be most in trouble. Families were considered to be in trouble if they found it more difficult to obtain care than they had in the past; someone in the family had been refused care for financial reasons; the family had needed care and not gotten it (in general, for special services or in response to a serious illness); or such an illness had caused the family major financial problems.

Applying these criteria, we can conclude that 14 percent (or almost 10 million families) may be considered to be in trouble. These families are most heavily represented among poor minorities (29%), the unemployed (26%), the publicly insured (20%) or those with no coverage (28%). This summary index bears out the profile of who is most in need drawn from the individual indicators discussed earlier in this chapter.

As suggested in earlier chapters, though the provision of medical care to traditionally disadvantaged groups has improved significantly over the past two decades, inequities do remain. A substantial number of American families can be considered "in trouble," based on both traditional and more problem-oriented indicators of access. Health policy should address the impact of cost containment strategies on the access of these people in particular, as the data just presented demonstrate the central importance of financial barriers in impeding access to required services for these groups. The next chapter will provide an overview of the findings in this and previous chapters and the implications of these results for new health policy alternatives in this cost-containment oriented decade of the 80s.

**TABLE 4.1 Percent of U.S. Families Who Found It More Difficult to Get Medical Help Relative to Those Who Found It Easier: 1982**

SPECIAL ACCESS PROBLEMS: MORE DIFFICULT TO GET MEDICAL HELP (a)

| POPULATION SUBGROUPS | Percent Who Found It More Difficult | Percent Who Found It Easier | Net Percent Who Found It More Difficult |
|---|---|---|---|
| RESIDENCE | | | |
| SMSA | | | |
| Central City | 6 | 4 | 2 |
| Other | 6 | 4 | 2 |
| Non SMSA | 6 | 5 | 1 |
| Non Farm | 5 | 4 | 1 |
| Farm | 9 | 6 | 3 |
| FAMILY INCOME | | | |
| Low | 8 | 5 | 3 |
| Medium | 5 | 5 | 0 |
| High | 4 | 4 | 0 |
| ETHNICITY | | | |
| Hispanic | 10 | 7 | 3 |
| Non Hispanic | | | |
| White | 5 | 3 | 2 |
| Black | 10 | 11 | -1 |
| 150% POVERTY LEVEL | | | |
| BY RACE | | | |
| Poor | | | |
| White | 10 | 6 | 4 |
| Nonwhite | 9 | 5 | 4 |
| Non Poor | | | |
| White | 13 | 10 | 3 |
| White | 4 | 3 | 1 |
| Nonwhite | 8 | 11 | -3 |
| MAIN EARNER | | | |
| EMPLOYMENT STATUS | | | |
| Employed | 5 | 5 | 0 |
| Not employed | 17 | 5 | 12 |
| Not in labor force | 6 | 3 | 3 |
| INSURANCE COVERAGE | | | |
| Private only | 5 | 5 | 0 |
| Public only | 8 | 4 | 4 |
| Public and private | 4 | 3 | 1 |
| No insurance | 16 | 5 | 11 |
| TOTAL | 6 | 4 | 2 |

(a) Percent table N is of U. S. families equals 96; percent NA equals 4.

**TABLE 4.2  Percent of U.S. Families Who Had Financial Problems Associated with Illness: 1982**

SPECIAL ACCESS PROBLEMS:  FINANCIAL PROBLEMS ASSOCIATED WITH ILLNESS

| POPULATION SUBGROUPS | Percent for Whom Earnings Were Reduced Due to Illness (a) | Percent of Families With Reduced Earnings for Whom This Was Serious (b) | Percent Refused Care For Financial Reasons (a) |
|---|---|---|---|
| RESIDENCE | | | |
| SMSA | | | |
| Central City | 5 | 33 | 2 |
| Other | 5 | 38 | 2 |
| Non SMSA | 5 | 30 | 1 |
| Non Farm | 5 | 26 | 1 |
| Farm | 4 | 28 | 2 |
| FAMILY INCOME | | - | |
| Low | 6 | 48 | 2 |
| Medium | 6 | 20 | 1 |
| High | 3 | 9 | 1 |
| ETHNICITY | | | |
| Hispanic | 6 | 31 | 3 |
| Non Hispanic | | | |
| White | 5 | 32 | 1 |
| Black | 5 | 30 | 2 |
| 150% POVERTY LEVEL | | | |
| BY RACE | | | |
| Poor | 7 | 50 | 3 |
| White | 8 | 49 | 3 |
| Nonwhite | 5 | 61 | 3 |
| Non Poor | 4 | 21 | 1 |
| White | 4 | 23 | 1 |
| Nonwhite | | - | 1 |
| MAIN EARNER | | | |
| EMPLOYMENT STATUS | | | |
| Employed | 5 | 23 | 1 |
| Not employed | 5 | 46 | 4 |
| Not in labor force | 6 | 54 | 2 |
| INSURANCE COVERAGE | | | |
| Private only | 5 | 25 | 1 |
| Public only | 5 | 67 | 4 |
| Public and private | 5 | 41 | 1 |
| No insurance | 7 | 57 | 4 |
| | | | |
| TOTAL | 5 | 32 | 2 |

- Indicates estimate based on fewer than 25 unweighted observations.
(a) Percent table N is of U.S. families equals 99; percent NA equals 1.
(b) Percent table N is of U.S. families equals 5; percent with earnings not reduced, NA equals 95.

**TABLE 4.3  Percent of U.S. Adults Whose Insurance Coverage Changed in the Last Year: 1982**

| POPULATION SUBGROUPS | Percent Whose Coverage Changed (a) | Percent of Changes in Which Coverage Was More | Percent of Changes in Which Coverage Was Less(b) | Net More(+)/Less(-) | SPECIAL ACCESS PROBLEMS: Percent With Less Coverage Who Were Unable to Get Care (c) | CHANGES IN INSURANCE COVERAGE: Percent With Less Coverage Who Had to Change Their Regular Source (c) | Percent With Less Coverage Who Put Off Care (c) |
|---|---|---|---|---|---|---|---|
| **AGE** | | | | | | | |
| 18-34 | 21 | 43 | 26 | 17 | 10 | 13 | 28 |
| 35-54 | 25 | 42 | 25 | 17 | 7 | 5 | 22 |
| 55-64 | 21 | 30 | 34 | -4 | 17 | 11 | 22 |
| 65+ | 17 | 30 | 19 | 11 | 2 | 12 | 7 |
| **RESIDENCE** | | | | | | | |
| SMSA | 21 | 41 | 24 | 17 | 10 | 10 | 26 |
| Central City | 19 | 35 | 26 | 9 | 12 | 13 | 34 |
| Other | 22 | 44 | 23 | 21 | 8 | 9 | 22 |
| Non SMSA | 23 | 32 | 29 | 3 | 10 | 10 | 16 |
| Non Farm | 24 | 33 | 30 | 3 | 10 | 10 | 15 |
| Farm | 15 | 22 | 19 | 3 | - | - | - |
| **FAMILY INCOME** | | | | | | | |
| Low | 17 | 30 | 29 | 1 | 18 | 11 | 20 |
| Medium | 22 | 45 | 22 | 23 | 10 | 14 | 34 |
| High | 25 | 40 | 25 | 15 | 4 | 8 | 20 |
| **ETHNICITY** | | | | | | | |
| Hispanic | 23 | 42 | 30 | 12 | - | - | 33 |
| Non Hispanic | | | | | | | |
| White | 22 | 38 | 25 | 13 | 9 | 9 | 23 |
| Black | 16 | 42 | 32 | 10 | 4 | 6 | 14 |
| **150% POVERTY LEVEL** | | | | | | | |
| **BY RACE** | | | | | | | |
| Poor | 14 | 24 | 37 | -13 | 23 | 14 | 23 |
| White | 17 | 25 | 34 | -9 | 25 | 12 | 24 |
| Nonwhite | 8 | 22 | 52 | -30 | 11 | 19 | 22 |
| Non Poor | 23 | 41 | 24 | 17 | 6 | 9 | 23 |
| White | 23 | 41 | 23 | 18 | 7 | 10 | 24 |
| Nonwhite | 22 | 41 | 26 | 15 | - | - | - |
| **MAIN EARNER** | | | | | | | |
| **EMPLOYMENT STATUS** | | | | | | | |
| Employed | 22 | 43 | 24 | 19 | 8 | 10 | 24 |
| Not employed | 19 | 24 | 37 | -13 | 25 | 7 | 23 |
| Not in labor force | 18 | 22 | 28 | -6 | 12 | 13 | 20 |
| **INSURANCE COVERAGE** | | | | | | | |
| Private only | 23 | 43 | 23 | 20 | 6 | 8 | 21 |
| Public only | 18 | 8 | 39 | -31 | 21 | 23 | 15 |
| Public and private | 20 | 38 | 18 | 20 | 4 | 7 | 18 |
| No insurance | 10 | 0 | 83 | -83 | 36 | 23 | 36 |
| **TOTAL** | 21 | 39 | 26 | 13 | 10 | 10 | 23 |

- Indicates estimate based on fewer than 25 unweighted observations.
(a) Percent table N is of U.S. adults equals 93; percent NA equals 7. Respondents may have reported more than one way in which their coverage changed. Hence, the percentages reflect the number of times that type of change was given as a proportion of the number of all changes reported.
(b) Percent table N is of U.S. adults equals 18; percent with no change, NA equals 82.
(c) Percent table N is of U.S. adults equals 5; percent whose coverage not dropped or reduced, NA equals 95.

**TABLE 4.4 Percent of U.S. Families Who Needed Care but Did Not Get It: 1982**

SPECIAL ACCESS PROBLEMS: NEEDED CARE BUT DID NOT GET IT

| POPULATION SUBGROUPS | Percent Who Needed Care But Did Not Get It (a) | Percent Who Tried of Those Who Needed Care But Did Not Get It (b) |
|---|---|---|
| RESIDENCE | | |
| SMSA | 6 | 38 |
| Central City | 6 | 40 |
| Other | 6 | 37 |
| Non SMSA | 5 | 46 |
| Non Farm | 4 | 49 |
| Farm | 6 | - |
| FAMILY INCOME | | |
| Low | 8 | 38 |
| Medium | 4 | 38 |
| High | 4 | 45 |
| ETHNICITY | | |
| Hispanic | 9 | 31 |
| Non Hispanic | | |
| White | 5 | 39 |
| Black | 8 | 49 |
| 150% POVERTY LEVEL | | |
| BY RACE | | |
| Poor | 9 | 40 |
| White | 8 | 37 |
| Nonwhite | 11 | 48 |
| Non Poor | 4 | 40 |
| White | 4 | 38 |
| Nonwhite | 6 | - |
| MAIN EARNER | | |
| EMPLOYMENT STATUS | | |
| Employed | 6 | 41 |
| Not employed | 11 | 20 |
| Not in labor force | 5 | 46 |
| INSURANCE COVERAGE | | |
| Private only | 5 | 39 |
| Public only | 8 | 49 |
| Public and private | 4 | 37 |
| No insurance | 15 | 38 |
| TOTAL | 6 | 40 |

-Indicates estimate based on fewer than 25 unweighted observations.
(a) Percent table N is of U.S. families equals 99; NA equals 1.
(b) Percent table N is of U.S. families equals 5; percent who did get care when needed. NA equals 95.

**TABLE 4.5  Reasons U.S. Families Who Needed Care Did Not Get It When They Tried or Did Not Try: 1982**

| REASONS DID NOT GET CARE WHEN TRIED OR DID NOT TRY | PERCENTAGE | |
|---|---|---|
| | Tried (a) | Did Not Try (b) |
| Could not get an appointment | 10% | - |
| Did not know a good doctor | 11 | 4 |
| Cost too much | 33 | 59 |
| Not covered by insurance | 19 | 11 |
| Other reasons | 27 | 26 |
| TOTAL | 100% | 100% |

(a) Percent table N is of U.S. families equals 2; percent who did get care when needed or did not try. NA equals 98.
(b) Percent table N is of U.S. families equals 3; percent who did get care when needed, tried and did not get. NA equals 97.

**TABLE 4.6  Percent of U.S. Families Who Needed Special Services but Did Not Get Them: 1982**

SPECIAL ACCESS PROBLEMS: NEEDED SPECIAL SERVICES BUT DID NOT GET THEM

| POPULATION SUBGROUPS | Percent Who Needed Special Services But Did Not Get Them (a) |
|---|---|
| RESIDENCE | |
| SMSA | |
|   Central City | 6 |
|   Other | 5 |
| Non SMSA | 6 |
|   Non Farm | 3 |
|   Farm | 2 |
| FAMILY INCOME | |
|   Low | 5 |
|   Medium | 5 |
|   High | 5 |
| ETHNICITY | |
|   Hispanic | 3 |
|   Non Hispanic | |
|     White | 5 |
|     Black | 7 |
| 150% POVERTY LEVEL | |
| BY RACE | |
|   Poor | 6 |
|     White | 5 |
|     Nonwhite | 10 |
|   Non Poor | 5 |
|     White | 4 |
|     Nonwhite | 6 |
| MAIN EARNER EMPLOYMENT STATUS | |
|   Employed | 5 |
|   Not employed | 8 |
|   Not in labor force | 3 |
| INSURANCE COVERAGE | |
|   Private only | 5 |
|   Public only | 6 |
|   Public and private | 3 |
|   No insurance | 8 |
| TOTAL | 5 |

(a) Percent table N is of U.S. families equals 97; percent NA equals 3.

95

**TABLE 4.7 Percent of U.S. Families with Seriously Ill Family Member: 1982**

SPECIAL ACCESS PROBLEMS: SERIOUSLY ILL FAMILY MEMBER

| POPULATION SUBGROUPS | Percent With Seriously Ill Family Member(a) | Percent of Families With Serious Illness Who Needed Help At Home(b) | Percent of Families With Serious Illness in Which There Were Major Personal Changes(b) | Percent of Families With Serious Illness Who Were Not Able to Obtain Special Services(b) | Percent of Families With Serious Illness For Whom It Was Major Financial Problem(b) |
|---|---|---|---|---|---|
| RESIDENCE | | | | | |
| SMSA | 10 | 15 | 14 | 11 | 22 |
| Central City | 9 | 14 | 15 | 14 | 28 |
| Other | 10 | 16 | 13 | 9 | 18 |
| Non SMSA | 8 | 23 | 14 | 12 | 25 |
| Non Farm | 9 | 24 | 15 | 14 | 27 |
| Farm | - | - | - | - | - |
| FAMILY INCOME | | | | | |
| Low | 11 | 17 | 14 | 16 | 34 |
| Medium | 7 | 16 | 13 | 8 | 17 |
| High | 8 | 16 | 14 | 6 | 8 |
| ETHNICITY | | | | | |
| Hispanic | 11 | 19 | 9 | 11 | 39 |
| Non Hispanic | | | | | |
| White | 9 | 17 | 15 | 9 | 18 |
| Black | 11 | 16 | 11 | 24 | 40 |
| 150% POVERTY LEVEL | | | | | |
| BY RACE | | | | | |
| Poor | 11 | 20 | 15 | 18 | 38 |
| White | 11 | 21 | 15 | 15 | 34 |
| Nonwhite | 13 | 19 | 13 | 26 | 50 |
| Non Poor | 8 | 15 | 13 | 8 | 15 |
| White | 9 | 16 | 14 | 7 | 14 |
| Nonwhite | 8 | - | - | - | - |
| MAIN EARNER | | | | | |
| EMPLOYMENT STATUS | | | | | |
| Employed | 7 | 14 | 12 | 7 | 20 |
| Not employed | 11 | 17 | 24 | 3 | 29 |
| Not in labor force | 16 | 21 | 16 | 17 | 26 |
| INSURANCE COVERAGE | | | | | |
| Private only | 7 | 13 | 14 | 8 | 18 |
| Public only | 17 | 43 | 21 | 26 | 36 |
| Public and private | 15 | 17 | 11 | 11 | 16 |
| No insurance | 8 | 17 | 23 | 7 | 52 |
| TOTAL | 9 | 17 | 14 | 11 | 22 |

- Indicates estimate based on fewer than 25 unweighted observations.
(a) Percent table N is of U.S. families equals 99; percent NA equals 1.
(b) Percent table N is of U.S. families equals 9; percent with no seriously ill member. NA equals 91.

SPECIAL ACCESS PROBLEMS: MEDICAL EMERGENCY IN THE YEAR

| Population Subgroups | Percent with Medical Emergency (a) | Location of Visit for Medical Emergency (b) | | | | | Percent with Medical Emergency Who Had Problems in Getting There (b) |
|---|---|---|---|---|---|---|---|
| | | Doctor's Office or HMO | Hospital or ER | OPD | Other Place | Didn't Go Anywhere | |
| **AGE** | | | | | | | |
| 1–5 | 22 | 17 | 78 | | 4 | 1 | 3 |
| 6–17 | 15 | 15 | 79 | | 6 | 0 | 5 |
| 18–34 | 16 | 14 | 81 | | 5 | 1 | 4 |
| 35–54 | 14 | 16 | 79 | | 4 | 0 | 9 |
| 55–64 | 12 | 28 | 70 | | 2 | 1 | 3 |
| 65+ | 11 | 27 | 71 | | 1 | 2 | 1 |
| **RESIDENCE** | | | | | | | |
| SMSA | 16 | 17 | 79 | | 4 | 1 | 4 |
| Central City | 16 | 18 | 77 | | 5 | 0 | 3 |
| Other | 15 | 16 | 80 | | 4 | 1 | 5 |
| Non SMSA | 13 | 18 | 77 | | 5 | 0 | 7 |
| Non Farm | 13 | 17 | 79 | | 4 | 0 | 8 |
| Farm | 13 | 24 | 67 | | 8 | 0 | 3 |
| **FAMILY INCOME** | | | | | | | |
| Low | 16 | 16 | 78 | | 5 | 1 | 5 |
| Medium | 14 | 16 | 77 | | 6 | 1 | 2 |
| High | 14 | 19 | 78 | | 3 | 0 | 6 |
| **ETHNICITY** | | | | | | | |
| Hispanic | 18 | 11 | 86 | | 3 | 0 | 2 |
| Non Hispanic | | | | | | | |
| White | 14 | 19 | 76 | | 4 | 1 | 5 |
| Black | 16 | 12 | 85 | | 3 | 0 | 4 |
| **150% POVERTY LEVEL BY RACE** | | | | | | | |
| Poor | 16 | 10 | 83 | | 6 | 1 | 5 |
| White | 16 | 12 | 81 | | 5 | 2 | 6 |
| Nonwhite | 19 | 6 | 87 | | 8 | 0 | 2 |
| Non Poor | 14 | 19 | 77 | | 4 | 0 | 5 |
| White | 15 | 20 | 76 | | 4 | 0 | 5 |
| Nonwhite | 13 | 17 | 80 | | 3 | 0 | 6 |
| **MAIN EARNER EMPLOYMENT STATUS** | | | | | | | |
| Employed | 15 | 17 | 78 | | 4 | 0 | 5 |
| Not employed | 16 | 10 | 84 | | 5 | 0 | 2 |
| Not in labor force | 16 | 21 | 74 | | 4 | 2 | 6 |
| **INSURANCE COVERAGE** | | | | | | | |
| Private only | 15 | 15 | 80 | | 4 | 0 | 5 |
| Public only | 14 | 13 | 73 | | 8 | 6 | 5 |
| Public and private | 15 | 18 | 79 | | 3 | 0 | 2 |
| No insurance | 14 | 22 | 73 | | 5 | 0 | 6 |
| **TOTAL** | 15 | 17 | 77 | | 4 | 1 | 5 |

(a) Percent table N is of U.S. population equals 99; percent NA equals 1.
(b) Percent table N is of U.S. population equals 14; percent without a medical emergency, NA equals 86.

**TABLE 4.9 Percent of U.S. Population with Medical Emergency in the Year Who Are Not At All Satisfied with Care Received: 1982**

SPECIAL ACCESS PROBLEMS: NOT AT ALL SATISFIED WITH CARE RECEIVED (a)

| | Travel Time | Office Waiting Time | Time With Doctor | Information Provided | Out-of-Pocket Cost | Quality of Care | Visit Overall |
|---|---|---|---|---|---|---|---|
| **AGE** | | | | | | | |
| 1-5 | 6 | 23 | 11 | 14 | 16 | 13 | 12 |
| 6-17 | 6 | 19 | 8 | 8 | 17 | 5 | 8 |
| 18-34 | 8 | 25 | 15 | 22 | 24 | 16 | 16 |
| 35-54 | 5 | 19 | 10 | 14 | 10 | 7 | 8 |
| 55-64 | 2 | 11 | 6 | 8 | 8 | 10 | 8 |
| 65+ | 2 | 4 | 4 | 11 | 12 | 4 | 3 |
| **RESIDENCE** | | | | | | | |
| SMSA | 6 | 20 | 11 | 16 | 17 | 11 | 12 |
|   Central City | 7 | 24 | 9 | 16 | 16 | 9 | 9 |
|   Other | 5 | 17 | 13 | 16 | 18 | 12 | 13 |
| Non SMSA | 6 | 19 | 8 | 11 | 15 | 8 | 9 |
|   Non Farm | 7 | 20 | 10 | 13 | 15 | 10 | 10 |
|   Farm | 3 | 17 | 2 | 5 | 14 | 2 | 4 |
| **FAMILY INCOME** | | | | | | | |
| Low | 7 | 21 | 13 | 15 | 24 | 14 | 14 |
| Medium | 5 | 13 | 9 | 14 | 15 | 7 | 8 |
| High | 6 | 23 | 10 | 15 | 11 | 10 | 10 |
| **ETHNICITY** | | | | | | | |
| Hispanic | 1 | 30 | 15 | 14 | 25 | 20 | 17 |
| Non Hispanic | | | | | | | |
|   White | 6 | 17 | 10 | 15 | 14 | 10 | 11 |
|   Black | 7 | 26 | 13 | 14 | 23 | 8 | 7 |
| **150% POVERTY LEVEL BY RACE** | | | | | | | |
| Poor | 9 | 24 | 14 | 15 | 24 | 13 | 14 |
|   White | 11 | 24 | 16 | 17 | 23 | 14 | 16 |
|   Nonwhite | 4 | 26 | 8 | 9 | 28 | 8 | 7 |
| Non Poor | 5 | 18 | 10 | 15 | 14 | 10 | 10 |
|   White | 5 | 18 | 9 | 14 | 14 | 9 | 10 |
|   Nonwhite | 9 | 27 | 20 | 20 | 17 | 13 | 10 |
| **MAIN EARNER EMPLOYMENT STATUS** | | | | | | | |
| Employed | 6 | 22 | 12 | 16 | 18 | 12 | 12 |
| Not employed | 4 | 23 | 3 | 20 | 20 | 6 | 4 |
| Not in labor force | 4 | 9 | 7 | 11 | 10 | 7 | 7 |
| **INSURANCE COVERAGE** | | | | | | | |
| Private only | 6 | 20 | 11 | 13 | 16 | 10 | 10 |
| Public only | 10 | 18 | 8 | 8 | 15 | 13 | 16 |
| Public and private | 2 | 17 | 5 | 23 | 10 | 9 | 8 |
| No insurance | 9 | 26 | 20 | 22 | 31 | 15 | 19 |
| **TOTAL** | 6 | 20 | 11 | 15 | 16 | 10 | 11 |

(a) Percent table N is of U.S. population equals 14; percent without a medical emergency. NA equals 86.

98

**TABLE 4.10 Percent of U.S. Families in Trouble, Based on Access Summary Measure: 1982**

SPECIAL ACCESS PROBLEMS: U.S. FAMILIES IN TROUBLE

| POPULATION SUBGROUPS | Percent of U.S. Families in Trouble (a) |
|---|---|
| RESIDENCE | |
| SMSA | 15 |
| Central City | 15 |
| Other | 15 |
| Non SMSA | 12 |
| Non Farm | 12 |
| Farm | 14 |
| FAMILY INCOME | |
| Low | 18 |
| Medium | 12 |
| High | 11 |
| ETHNICITY | |
| Hispanic | 21 |
| Non Hispanic | |
| White | 13 |
| Black | 22 |
| 150% POVERTY LEVEL | |
| BY RACE | |
| Poor | 21 |
| White | 19 |
| Nonwhite | 29 |
| Non Poor | 12 |
| White | 12 |
| Nonwhite | 18 |
| MAIN EARNER | |
| EMPLOYMENT STATUS | |
| Employed | 14 |
| Not employed | 26 |
| Not in labor force | 14 |
| INSURANCE COVERAGE | |
| Private only | 13 |
| Public only | 20 |
| Public and private | 12 |
| No insurance | 28 |
| TOTAL | 14 |

(a) Percent table N is of U. S. families equals 100.

# Chapter 5
## Summary and Implications

This study was undertaken to measure current levels of access to medical care in the United States and to better understand some of the reasons why access differs according to social and economic characteristics of the population. Specific questions it addresses include:

1) Have steady improvements in the access of traditionally disadvantaged groups such as minorities and the poor documented through the decades of the 50s, 60s and 70s continued into the 80s?

2) Are there special access problems associated with chronic illness, medical emergencies and other serious conditions which traditional measures of access, such as overall physician visits and hospital days, fail to reveal?

3) Have the recession and high unemployment rates of recent years accompanied by cutbacks in public health care programs and private insurance coverage stymied or reversed the improving access trends of earlier periods and caused new problems in getting medical care for major sectors of the population?

4) What are the implications of the findings for achieving or maintaining equity of access to medical care in the face of increasing constraints on the economy and the health care delivery system?

This chapter summarizes key findings from previous chapters and discusses their implications for future policies about the distribution of health care. We will consider each of the major dimensions of potential and realized access to medical care separately.

The potential dimensions include: 1) the presence and characteristics of a person's regular source of care; 2) the convenience of services received; and 3) the ability of people to pay for their medical care. The realized dimensions of access are: 1) actual use of physician, hospital and preventive services; 2) whether people get services when they perceive a need for care; and 3) satisfaction with services received.

The discussion of each dimension of access will highlight trends, the current situation and what the future may hold. We will consider the situation for the country as a whole as well as for subgroups of special interest defined according to age, residence, income, ethnicity, employment and insurance coverage. This review of the findings is of necessity selective, given the many facts presented in the previous chapters. It attempts to focus on those most relevant for policy options to achieve equity of access to medical care.

## Potential Access

### Regular source of care

About 90 percent of the population have a regular source of care. The proportion has not changed substantially since the early 1970s. Children and the elderly are most likely to have a regular source. When we control for other factors, we find no significant differences in the proportion of people who do not have a regular source of care according to ethnicity, income or residence, nor do we find that people in families where the main earner is unemployed fare worse than the employed. Further, illness and disability are not significant determinants of who has a regular source of care. Thus, it is unlikely that the influence of having a regular source of care on other dimensions of access discussed in subsequent sections can be explained as a selection effect. People without a regular source of care are not less likely to see a physician only because they are less ill and do not need a physician. Rather, not having a regular source of care directly influences whether people will see a doctor, as well as other measures of access independent of need for medical care.

People are less likely to have a regular source of care if they have moved into the community recently, do not have health insurance, live in large families or are male. The most mutable policy-relevant variable among these is health insurance. Some 20 million people do not have health insurance and over one-fifth of these (more than four million) do not have a regular source of care. As we have observed in the previous chapters and will see throughout this review of the major dimensions of access, those without insurance are perhaps the most readily identified disadvantaged segment of the population with respect to both potential and realized access to care.

Identifying a particular physician as a regular source of care may promote continuity of care, a preventive emphasis, open provider-patient communications and patient compliance with a medical regimen. More than three-quarters of the population and 87 percent of those with a regular source of care identify a particular physician. The proportion who identify a particular practitioner has declined slightly in the past ten to fifteen years. A shift from solo practice and partnerships to larger group practices and health maintenance organizations as well as use of outpatient departments and emergency rooms and, more recently, "emergicenters" may account for reduced patient identification with a particular physician.

Groups least likely to identify with a particular physician include the uninsured or publicly insured, those who have recently moved and males. In addition, central city residents and poor nonwhites are more likely to have a regular place but no particular provider they see there. About one-fourth of the poor nonwhites (around 3.5 million) fall into this category. One reason is that they are the most likely of all major population groups examined to use outpatient departments or emergency rooms as their regular source of care.

Growing impersonality may be a price that must be paid as more ambulatory care is provided by larger organizations and less by solo practitioners. However, large organization sponsorship of ambulatory care does not necessarily mean lack of identification with a particular provider. Both the Community Hospital Group Practice Program and the Municipal Health Services Program are examples of hospital and city-sponsored primary care programs that provide inner city and poor patients with more personalized forms of care in which they may go to particular providers in those settings (Aday, et al., 1984; Andersen, et al., 1982).

## Convenience of care

The rationale for including convenience as a major potential access dimension is that the ease of obtaining service and, conversely, the difficulties, not only give us a way of rating current system performance but also help us to explain resultant realized access measures—actual use of and satisfaction with health care services.

In 1982, 83 percent of the population reported waiting times of 30 minutes or less at their last visit. Our earlier studies are not completely comparable since we asked about usual waiting time at the regular source of care. Still, the proportion reporting waiting times of 30 minutes or less was 56 percent in 1970 and 64 percent in 1976 (Aday, et al., 1980: 66), suggesting a trend toward reduced waiting time. This may reflect the increasing supply of physicians and greater efforts to respond to patient wants.

The groups with the longest waits are Hispanics, Blacks, poor nonwhites and those who use a hospital out-patient department or emergency room or have no regular source of care. These groups, along with central city and rural residents, have traditionally had longer waits than the rest of the population, but the differences appear to be decreasing over time (Aday, et al., 1980: 66–67).

Still, in 1982 twelve percent of the poor nonwhite group reported a wait of one hour or more compared to five percent for the population as a whole. What is an "appropriate" or acceptable distribution for waiting times in the country? How important is waiting time compared to other realized measures of access? Such questions are not easily answered. We do know that patients are concerned about waiting times, and a wait of an hour or more would seem to exceed almost any commonly accepted norm of "appropriate" access. Although total equity has not been attained, waiting times are becoming more standardized. Providing those who use a hospital outpatient facility or have no regular source with an identified practitioner as a regular source would seem to go a long way in reducing the remaining inequity.

Do hard times exacerbate inconveniences in obtaining medical care? About one-quarter of the people living in families in which the main earner was unemployed had waits in the doctor's office of over 30 minutes compared to 16 percent for individuals in families with an employed main wage earner. Further, six percent of U.S. families found it more difficult to get medical help in the last year compared to four percent who found it easier. The poor, particularly the unemployed and the uninsured, were more likely to report increased difficulty in getting medical care. Thus, we have some indication, but not overwhelming evidence, of increased inconvenience getting medical care in the 80s, especially for the more socioeconomically disadvantaged subgroups.

## Financing

Some means of paying for services either directly or through a third party is necessary for access to be realized. About one-tenth of the population (20 million people) reported no public or private health insurance in 1982. Since a similar proportion reported no insurance in 1976, economic conditions and changing eligibility for public programs did not appear to affect the overall proportion of people with insurance coverage (Aday and Andersen, 1984). Further, while the low income, those without a regular source and minority groups were somewhat less likely to be insured in both 1976 and 1982, the discrepancies between them and the rest of the population did not *increase* between 1976 and 1982.

In 1982, 21 percent of the adults reported their health insurance coverage changed in the last year. Actually, more of them reported an increase (39%) than a decrease (26%) in coverage. However, some of the traditionally disadvantaged groups did report *less* coverage, including 37 percent of the poor, 52 percent of poor nonwhites, 39 percent of those with public insurance only and 37 percent of the unemployed. These groups may well be the first to suffer the consequences of increasing fiscal constraint in the delivery of health care.

Nine percent of U.S. families reported at least one family member who had a "serious illness, was chronically sick or needed medical treatment or hospitalization fairly often." Twenty-two percent of these families reported a major financial problem as a result. Most likely to report major financial problems were the uninsured (52%), poor nonwhites (50%), Blacks (40%), Hispanics (39%) and people with public insurance only (36%). These perceptions point up the problems our system faces in buffering major segments of the population against the financial impact of serious illness.

Perhaps the most direct question asked about the impact of financial impediments to care in 1982 was "whether any family members had been refused health care in the past year because they lacked insurance and could not pay." Two percent of the families said "yes." While the percentage is small, it still represents almost 1.5 million families. Further, families with an unemployed main earner and those with public insurance or no insurance were twice as likely as the population as a whole to report such an occurrence.

Financial barriers to care remain greater for minorities, the poor, the uninsured and the publicly-insured. The evidence is not so clear as to whether these problems are getting worse. What is "tolerable" is again a political and ethical question. However, the results suggest the system continues to fall short of a goal to remove major financial barriers to care and protect *all* families against major financial hardships caused by illness.

## Realized access

### Use of services

Differences in the proportion seeing a physician traceable to ethnic or income factors have decreased continually since the 1950s, and have been practically eliminated by the 1980s. Further, being in a family with an unemployed main earner does not appear to be a major barrier to seeing a physician.

Seeing the physician today appears to be primarily a function of demographic variables—age and sex—and amount of disability, suggesting a system that is, by and large, "equitable." However, people without insurance, without a regular source of care or living on a farm are still less likely than the rest of the population to see a doctor. It does appear that providing additional coverage and entry to a regular source of care would bring the system even closer to equity. To expect such a policy to be adopted in the current political and economic climate, however, is probably not realistic.

The *number* of visits people receive once they present themselves to the doctor is largely explained by measures of illness. In addition, traditionally disadvantaged groups—the poor, minorities and those without insurance—actually have *more* visits than the rest of the population. However, once level of need is taken into account, these differences are largely eliminated, again suggesting a fairly equitable system. Even after adjustments are made for need and other factors, persons with public insurance coverage remain high utilizers of physician services, while those without a regular source of care appear to be low utilizers.

The proportion of the population hospitalized, like number of physician visits, suggests that the poor may actually be overutilizers. However, adjustments for illness level eliminates the apparent excess, suggesting they have more serious illness than the rest of the population. Being hospitalized is largely explained by need, again suggesting an equitable system. Two groups which stand out in contrast to such a general conclusion are the uninsured and those without a regular source of care. Even after adjustment for need and other factors, about six percent of both these groups are hospitalized compared to ten percent for the total population.

Preventive services for children (TB skin test, measles, DPT, and polio immunizations) show little variance by any of the demographic or enabling characteristics. This suggests an equitable system for children, at least for these variables. Preventive services for adults present a somewhat different picture. Blood pressure checks are less common for farm residents, the uninsured and those without a regular source of care, even after need and other factors are controlled for. Pap smears and breast examinations for females are less common in the same groups. In sum, preventive services for adults could probably be increased by expanding insurance coverage and primary care affiliations. However, as suggested in Chapter 2, external norms of appropriateness suggest that current utilization of some preventive services may already be above an acceptable level, calling into question the need for expansion in this area.

## Use relative to need

Possibly the measures of access most relevant to the idea of equity espoused here are those that directly relate use of services to perceived need. Six percent of the families in the U.S. (over four million) reported a member needed medical care in 1982 and did not get it. An all-too-familiar theme of limited access for certain sectors of the population is repeated here. Fifteen percent of uninsured families and eleven percent of poor nonwhite families and those with an unemployed main earner needed care and did not get it. The most common reason given for not getting needed care was that it cost too much.

More than six million families reported one or more

seriously ill members who needed frequent medical treatment. Eleven percent of these families looked for but were
unable to get special assistance in the last year such as
home care or admittance to a nursing home for the sick
person. The groups most likely to have such problems
(about 25 percent in each case) are Blacks, poor nonwhites
and those with public insurance only.

The examination of families who felt they needed care
and did not get it points out two parts of the access problem. Some people do not get care they feel they need for
the range of health problems most families face. They
often lack personal resources and are not covered by public
programs to enable them to obtain care. The reasons for
their inability to secure services are sometimes transitory
and reversible. Frequently we find the uninsured and the
unemployed in this group. Proposed policies to address
their needs (which have not been successfully implemented up to this point) have included federally spon-
sored health insurance linked to unemployment and coordinated efforts and pooling of risks by third party payers
to provide coverage for the uninsured.

Another, and probably smaller, group faces special access problems created by long-term chronic illness. They
may well have basic coverage from public or other sources.
However, it does not satisfy their special long-term needs,
and they do not have sufficient personal resources to make
up the deficit. The issue here is not so much extending
the kind of coverage generally found in our system, but
providing new benefits for long term problems. Groups
which appear especially in need of longer-term supports
include poor minorities and those covered through public
programs alone.

Most proposals to deal with both acute and chronic access problems require additional expenditure of public
funds. The current policies of fiscal constraint and concern

about budget deficits suggest such proposals will face significant barriers to approval and implementation.

## Satisfaction

One person in five was not completely satisfied with his or her last visit to a physician, and one in ten who had a medical emergency was not at all satisfied with care received in 1982. Apparently satisfaction has remained relatively high over time, with dissatisfaction about waiting time possibly of less concern now than in the past. This may reflect the increasing number of physicians and competition among providers to attract patients by reducing waiting times.

People are most likely to be less than completely satisfied with the out-of-pocket cost of care (four in ten), followed by waiting time (three in ten). Characteristics of the visit itself (time with the doctor, the information received, and the perceived quality of care) received the least criticism (about 20 percent.) The elderly are generally more satisfied with all aspects of their care than are other age groups. Farm residents tend to be more satisfied, and minority groups less satisfied than the public as a whole.

Satisfaction with office waiting time is less for people using outpatient departments and emergency rooms as their regular source of care. By far, actual waiting time is the most important factor in patient satisfaction with waiting time. While not surprising, this result does validate the association between satisfaction and the experience itself. Scheduling and office management practices that reduce waiting time do result in more satisfied patients.

Out-of-pocket cost is viewed as least satisfactory by persons with no insurance, while farm residents tend to be least critical. Evidence of the correlation between actual experience and satisfaction is shown again, since prices of visits tend to be less in rural areas, and people without insurance are apt to be most affected by out-of-pocket costs. No charges or minimum charges at the time of visit have traditionally been popular with consumers. Certainly, this aspect of HMO care has been attractive to enrollees. The recent growth of HMO enrollment is probably reinforced by the attractiveness of first dollar coverage for doctor visits.

Satisfaction with the overall quality of care reflects stable and positive relationships with providers. People who use a particular provider as a regular source of care, are long-time residents of their community, are in good health (possibly associating their health with their source of care), and are most satisfied with the quality of their care. We also know that patients tend to rate quality of care high when a physician spent time with them, gave them ample information about their illnesses and showed concern about their overall well-being (Andersen, et al., 1981). A policy which integrates personalized service with potential cost savings achieved through more bureaucratic forms of delivery, such as HMOs, provides a major challenge and opportunity to the medical care delivery system today.

In general, satisfaction with care levels is high by most standards today and does not appear to be declining. While the majority of the population believes there are major problems with the health care system as a whole (RWJF, 1983), they are much more satisfied with their own care. The latter perceptions are the ones we believe should be given more attention by policymakers. Still, levels of dissatisfaction are sufficiently high and correlated with experience in receiving medical care to justify continued monitoring. They are important in assessing how the system is performing and in suggesting new directions in delivery and finance.

## Summary: equity and its import for health policy

The following conclusions might be drawn about the major study questions posed at the beginning of this chapter.

1) Improvements in access to medical care for traditionally disadvantaged groups documented in earlier decades largely continued into the 1980s. The poor, minority groups and central city and farm residents mostly maintained their earlier gains or improved in relation to the rest of the population with respect to having a usual source of care or using hospital, physician and preventive services. However, some problems remain for these disadvantaged groups. They are less likely to go to a particular practitioner; more likely to use an outpatient department or emergency room as a regular source of care; and wait longer on average to see a physician. The most disadvantaged groups on most measures of access are the uninsured and those without a regular source of care.

2) The traditional access measures fail to reveal the problems of people with medical emergencies or serious chronic illness in the family. Support in securing care for long-term serious illness seems particularly limited for the disadvantaged groups (the poor, minorities and the publicly insured).

3) It is difficult to show the impact of the recession and medical care cutbacks in the trend data on traditional access measures. However, questions asked in 1982 about special problems in getting medical care indicate some people are certainly being adversely affected. They include the unemployed (and there were more of them than in any time since the Depression), the uninsured, racial minorities and the poor.

4) The country has come a long way toward achieving equity, measured in terms of services being primarily allocated on the basis of need. Further, the momentum

toward equity did not appear to have been substantially diminished by 1982. Still, serious access problems remained for some groups, and these problems were exacerbated by the recession and constraints on federal and local spending for medical care. Mounting budget deficits and efforts to cut costs make health care programs vulnerable, particularly in the public sector. Access to medical care should be closely monitored as financing and delivery programs are altered or cut back. The costs of such programs in terms of reduced access as well as the benefits of reduced spending need to be fully specified to inform future health care planning.

# References

Aday, Lu Ann and Ronald Andersen. *Development of Indices of Access to Medical Care.* Ann Arbor, MI: Health Administration Press. 1975.

——————. "Insurance Coverage and Access: Implications for Health Policy." *Health Services Research* 13 (Winter 1978): 369–77.

——————. "Equity of Access to Medical Care: A Conceptual and Empirical Overview." *Medical Care* 19 (December supplement 1981): 4–27.

——————. "The National Profile of Access to Medical Care: Where Do We Stand?" *American Journal of Public Health* 74 (1984): forthcoming.

Aday, Lu Ann et al. *Health Care in the U.S.: Equitable for Whom?* Beverly Hills, CA: Sage Publications. 1980.

——————. "II. Hospital-Sponsored Primary Care: Impact on Patient Access." *American Journal of Public Health* 74 (August 1984): 792–798.

Alpert, Joel J. et al. "Attitudes and Satisfaction of Low-Income Families Receiving Comprehensive Pediatric Care." *American Journal of Public Health* 60 (March 1970): 499–506.

American Academy of Pediatrics. *Your Child's Health.* Evanston, IL: American Academy of Pediatrics. 1983

American Cancer Society, Inc. *Guidelines for Cancer-Related Checkup: Recommendations and Rationale.* New York: American Cancer Society, Inc. 1980.

Andersen, Ronald. *A Behavioral Model of Families' Use of Health Services.* Research Series No. 25. Chicago, IL: Center for Health Administration Studies, University of Chicago. 1968.

Andersen, Ronald and Lu Ann Aday. "Access to Medical Care in the U.S.: Realized and Potential." *Medical Care* 16 (July 1978): 533–46.

Andersen, Ronald et al. "The Public's View as Input for Medical Manpower Planning." In R. A. Musacchio (ed.), *Socioeconomic Issues of Health.* Chicago, IL: American Medical Association. 1981.

——————. "Evaluating the Municipal Health Services Program." *Annals of the New York Academy of Sciences* 387 (May 21, 1982): 91–110.

Beck, R. G. and J. M. Horne. "Utilization of Publicly Insured Health Services in Saskatchewan Before, During and After Copayment." *Medical Care* 18 (August 1980): 787–806.

Becker, Marshall H. et al. "Predicting Mothers' Compliance with Pediatric Medical Regimens." *Journal of Pediatrics* 81 (October 1972): 843.

——————————. "A Field Experiment to Evaluate Various Outcomes of Continuity of Physician Care." *American Journal of Public Health* 64 (November 1974): 1062–70.

Berk, Aviva A. and Thomas C. Chalmers. "Cost and Efficacy of the Substitution of Ambulatory for Inpatient Care." *New England Journal of Medicine* 304 (February 12, 1981): 393–7.

Blendon, Robert J. et al. "An Era of Stress for Health Institutions: the 1980s." *Journal of the American Medical Association (JAMA)* 245 (May 8, 1981): 1843–5.

Breslau, Naomi. "Continuity Reexamined: Differential Impact on Satisfaction with Medical Care for Disabled and Normal Children." *Medical Care* 20 (April 1982): 347–59.

Breslau, Naomi and Edward A. Mortimer, Jr. "Seeing the Same Doctor: Determinants of Satisfaction with Specialty Care for Disabled Children." *Medical Care* 19 (July 1981): 741–58.

Breslau, Naomi and Kenneth G. Reeb. "Continuity of Care in a University-Based Practice." *Journal of Medical Education* 50 (1975): 965–9.

Breslow, Lester. "The Challenge to Health Statistics in the Eighties." *Public Health Reports* 96 (May–June 1981): 231–6.

Brook, R.H., et al. "Does Free Care Improve Adults' Health? Results from a Randomized Controlled Trial." *New England Journal of Medicine* 309 (December 8, 1983): 1426–34.

Canadian Task Force on the Periodic Health Examination. "The Periodic Health Examination." *Canadian Medical Journal* 121 (November 3, 1979): 1193–1254.

CHAS (Center for Health Administration Studies). "Evaluation of Municipal Health Services Program Phase I (Baseline) Study Report." (Report to the Health Care Financing Administration under contract HCFA 500-78-0097.) University of Chicago Center for Health Administration Studies. 1982.

Congressional Budget Office. *Changing the Structure of Medicare Benefits: Issues and Options.* Washington, DC: Congressional Budget Office. 1983.

Daniels, Norman. "Equity of Access to Health Care: Some Conceptual and Ethical Issues." *Milbank Memorial Fund Quarterly* 60 (Winter 1982): 51–81.

Davis, Karen and Roger Reynolds. "The Impact of Medicare and Medicaid on Access to Medical Care." In R. N. Rosett (ed.), *The Role of Health Insurance in the Health Services Sector.* New York: National Bureau of Economic Research. 1975.

Davis, Karen and Diane Rowland. "Uninsured and Underserved: Inequities in Health Care in the United States." *Milbank Memorial Fund Quarterly* 61 (Spring 1983): 149–76.

Davis, Karen et al. "Access to Health Care for the Poor: Does the Gap Remain?" *Annual Review of Public Health* 2 (1981): 159–82.

Department of Health and Human Services. *Health: United States, 1980.* DHHS Publication No. (PHS) 81–1232. Hyattsville, MD: Department of Health and Human Services. 1980.

Detmer, Don E. "Ambulatory Surgery." *New England Journal of Medicine* (305) (December 3, 1981): 1406–09.

Dutton, Diana B. and Ralph S. Silber. "Children's Health Outcomes in Six Different Ambulatory Care Delivery Systems." *Medical Care* 18 (July 1980): 693–714.

Egdahl, Richard H. "Physicians and the Containment of Health Care Costs." *New England Journal of Medicine* 304 (April 9, 1981): 900–01.

Enright, Sharon M. "Effect of Reaganomics on the U.S. Health Care System." *American Journal of Hospital Pharmacy* 39 (July 1982): 1169–75.

Enthoven, Alain C. *Health Plan: The Only Practical Solution to the Soaring Cost of Medical Care.* Reading, MA: Addison-Wesley. 1980.

—————. "The Competition Strategy: Status and Prospects." *New England Journal of Medicine* 304 (January 8, 1981): 109–112.

Estes, Carol L. "Austerity and Aging in the United States: 1980 and Beyond." *International Journal of Health Services* (December 4, 1982) 573–84.

Fein, Rashi. "Effects of Cost Sharing in Health Insurance." *New England Journal of Medicine* 305 (December 17, 1981): 1526–8.

Fleming, Gretchen V. "Hospital Structure and Consumer Satisfaction." *Health Services Research* 16 (Spring 1981): 43–63.

Foltz, Anne-Marie. *An Ounce of Prevention: Child Health Politics Under Medicaid.* Cambridge, MA: MIT Press. 1982

Freeborn, Donald K. and Merwyn R. Greenlick. "Evaluation of the Performance of Ambulatory Care Systems: Research Requirements and Opportunities." *Medical Care* 11 (January supplement, 1973): 68–75.

Freeman, Howard E. et al. "Community Health Centers: An Initiative of Enduring Utility." *Milbank Memorial Fund Quarterly* 60 (Spring 1982): 245–267.

Friedman, Emily. "Slicing the Pie Thinner: Hospitals and Physicians Square Off over Primary Care Services." *Hospitals, JAHA* 56 (October 16, 1982): 62–74.

Ginzberg, Eli. "Health Reform: The Outlook for the 1980s." *Inquiry* 15 (December 1978): 311–26.

——————. "The Competitive Solution: Two Views." *New England Journal of Medicine* 303 (November 26, 1980): 1112–5.

——————. "Cost Containment—Imaginary and Real." *New England Journal of Medicine* 308 (May 19, 1983): 1220–3.

Givens, Jimmie D. and Abigail J. Moss. "Redesigning the National Health Interview Survey's Data Collection Instrument." In *Silver Anniversary of the National Health Survey Act*. Hyattsville, MD: National Center for Health Statistics. 1981.

Goldman, Fred and Michael Grossman. "The Impact of Public Health Policy: The Case of Community Health Centers." Working Paper No. 1020. Cambridge, MA: National Bureau of Economic Research. 1982.

Gortmaker, Steven L. "Medicaid and the Health Care of Children in Poverty and Near Poverty: Some Successes and Failures." *Medical Care* 19 (June 1981): 567–82.

Gray, Alastair M. "Inequities in Health: The Black Report: A Summary and Comment." *International Journal of Health Services* 12 (3, 1982): 349–80.

Green, Lawrence W. et al. "Data Requirements to Measure Progress on the Objectives for the Nation in Health

Promotion and Disease Prevention." *American Journal of Public Health* 73 (January 1983): 18–24.

Gutmann, Amy. "For and Against Equal Access to Health Care." *Milbank Memorial Fund Quarterly* 59 (Summer 1981): 542–60.

Havighurst, Clark C. *Deregulating the Health Care Industry: Planning for Competition.* Cambridge, MA: Ballinger. 1982.

Heagarty, Margaret C. et al. "Some Comparative Costs in Comprehensive versus Fragmented Pediatric Care." *Pediatrics* 46 (1970): 596–603.

Hitt, David H. and Michael P. Harristhal. "Financing Health Care in the 1980s." *Hospitals, JAHA* 54 (January 1, 1980): 71–4.

Hollingsworth, J. Rogers. "Inequality in Levels of Health in England and Wales, 1891–1971." *Journal of Health and Social Behavior* 22 (September 1981): 268–83.

Hulka, Barbara S. "Epidemiological Applications to Health Services Research." *Journal of Community Health* 4 (Winter 1978): 140–9.

Hulka, Barbara S. et al. "Satisfaction with Medical Care in a Low-Income Population." *Journal of Chronic Disease* 24 (1971): 661–73.

Iglehart, John K. "The Administration Responds to the Cost Spiral." *New England Journal of Medicine* 305 (November 26, 1981): 1359–64.

[a]————. "Federal Policies and the Poor." *New England Journal of Medicine* 307 (September 23, 1982): 836–40.

[b]————. "The New Era of Prospective Pay-

ment for Hospitals." *New England Journal of Medicine* 307 (November 11, 1982): 1288–92.

——————. "Medicare Begins Prospective Payment of Hospitals." *New England Journal of Medicine* 308 (June 9, 1983): 1428–32.

Kasper, Judith A. and Gerald Barrish. "Usual Sources of Medical Care and their Characteristics." *Data Preview 12: NCHSR Health Care Expenditures Study.* DHHS Publication No. (PHS) 82–3324. Hyattsville, MD: National Center for Health Services Research. 1982.

Kasper, Judith A. and Marc L. Berk. "Waiting Times in Different Medical Settings: Appointment Waits and Office Waits." *Data Preview 6: NCHSR Health Care Expenditures Study.* DHHS Publication No. (PHS) 81–3296. Hyattsville, MD: National Center for Health Services Research. 1981.

Kasper, Judith A. et al. "Who Are the Uninsured?" *Data Preview 1: NCHSR Health Care Expenditures Study.* Hyattsville, MD: National Center for Health Services Research. 1980.

Kleinman, Joel C. et al. "Use of Ambulatory Medical Care by the Poor: Another Look at Equity." *Medical Care* 19 (October 1981): 1011–29.

Kovar, Mary G. "Health Status of U.S. Children and Use of Medical Care." *Public Health Reports* 97 (January–February 1982): 3–15.

Langwell, Kathryn M. and Sylvia F. Moore. "A Synthesis of Research on Competition in the Financing and Delivery of Health Services." *NCHSR Research Report Series.* DHHS Publication No. (PHS) 83–3327. Hyattsville, MD: National Center for Health Services Research. 1982.

Lewis, Charles et al. *A Right to Health: The Problem of Access to Primary Medical Care.* New York: John Wiley and Sons. 1976.

Lou Harris & Associates, Inc. *Access to Health Care Services in the United States: 1982.* New York: Lou Harris & Associates, Inc. 1982.

Luft, Harold S. *Health Maintenance Organizations: Dimensions of Performance.* New York: John Wiley and Sons. 1981.

——————————. "Health Maintenance Organizations and the Rationing of Medical Care." *Milbank Memorial Fund Quarterly* 60 (Spring 1982): 268–306.

Marcus, Alfred and Jeffrey D. Stone. "Racial/Ethnic Differences in Access to Health Care: Further Comments on the Use-Disability Ratio." *Medical Care* 20 (September 1982): 892–900.

Marks, Sylvia D. et al. "Ambulatory Surgery in an HMO: A Study of Costs, Quality of Care and Satisfaction." *Medical Care* 18 (February 1980): 127–46.

Master, Robert J. et al. "A Continuum of Care for the Inner City." *New England Journal of Medicine* 302 (June 26, 1980): 1434–40.

McNerney, Walter J. "Control of Health Care Costs in the 1980s." *New England Journal of Medicine* 303 (November 6, 1980): 1088–95.

Mechanic, David. "Some Dilemmas in Health Care Policy." *Milbank Memorial Fund Quarterly* 59 (Winter 1981): 1–15.

Melia, Edward P. et al. "Competition in the Health-Care Marketplace: A Beginning in California." *New England Journal of Medicine* 308 (March 31, 1983): 788–92.

Mindlin, Rowland L. and Paul M. Densen. "Medical Care of Urban Infants: Continuity of Care." *American Journal of Public Health* 59 (August, 1969): 1294–1301.

NCHS (National Center for Health Statistics). *Health: United States, 1980*. DHHS Publication No. (PHS) 81–1232. Washington, DC: Government Printing Office. 1980.

[a]_____. *Current Estimates from the National Health Interview Survey: United States, 1981*. DHHS Publication No. (PHS) 82–1569. Washington, DC: Government Printing Office. 1982.

[b]_____. *Health: United States, 1982*. DHHS Publication No. (PHS) 83–1232. Washington, DC: Government Printing Office. 1982.

_____. *Vital and Health Statistics: Physician Visits, United States, 1980*. DHHS Publication No. (PHS) 83–1572. Washington, DC: Government Printing Office. 1983.

Newachek, Paul W. et al. "Income and Illness." *Medical Care* 18 (December 1980): 1165–76.

Newhouse, Joseph P. et al. "Some Interim Results from a Controlled Trial of Cost Sharing in Health Insurance." *New England Journal of Medicine* 305 (December 17, 1981): 1501–7.

_____. *Some Interim Results from a Controlled Trial of Cost Sharing in Health Insurance*. R2847. Santa Monica, CA: Rand Corporation. 1982.

Office of the Assistant Secretary for Health: *Healthy People: The Surgeon General's Report on Health Promotion and Disease Prevention*. Stock No. 017-001-00416-2. Washington, DC: Government Printing Office. 1979.

Okada, Louise M. and Thomas T. H. Wan. "Impact of Community Health Centers and Medicaid on the Use of Health Services." *Public Health Reports* 95 (November–December 1980): 520–34.

Orr, Suezanne T. and C. Arden Miller. "Utilization of Health Services by Poor Children since Advent of Medicaid." *Medical Care* 19 (June 1981): 583–90.

Penchansky, Roy and J. William Thomas. "The Concept of Access: Definition and Relationship to Consumer Satisfaction." *Medical Care* 19 (February 1981): 127–40.

Pollitt, Christopher. "Corporate Rationalization of American Health Care: A Visitor's Appraisal." *Journal of Health Politics, Policy and Law* 7 (Spring 1982): 227–253.

President's Commission for the Study of Ethical Problems in Medicine and Biomedical and Behavioral Research. *Securing Access to Medical Care: The Ethical Implications of Differences in the Availability of Health Services. (Volume I: Report. Volume III: Appendices—Empirical, Legal and Conceptual Studies.)* Washington, DC: Government Printing Office. 1983.

Rice, Dorothy P. "Health Statistics: Past and Present." *New England Journal of Medicine* 305 (July 23, 1981): 219–20.

Robert Wood Johnson Foundation. *Special Report: Updated Report on Access to Health Care for the American People.* Princeton, NJ: Robert Wood Johnson Foundation. 1983.

Rogers, David E. et al. "Who Needs Medicaid?" *New England Journal of Medicine* 307 (July 1, 1982): 13–18.

Roos, Leslie L. et al. "Continuity of Care: Does It Contribute to Quality of Care?" *Medical Care* 18 (February 1980): 174–84.

Rosenblatt, Roger A. and Ira S. Moscovice. *Rural Health Care*. New York: John Wiley and Sons. 1982.

Sawyer, Darwin O. "Assessing Access Constraints on System Equity: Source of Care Differences in the Distribution of Medical Services." *Health Services Research* 17 (Spring 1982): 27–44.

Shortell, Stephen M. et al. "The Relationships Among Dimensions of Health Services in Two Provider Systems: A Causal Model Approach." *Journal of Health and Social Behavior* 18 (June 1977): 139–59.

Sloan, Frank and Judith D. Bentkover. *Access to Ambulatory Care and the U.S. Economy*. Lexington, MA: Lexington Books, 1979.

Snoke, Albert W. "What Good Is Legislation—Or Planning—If We Can't Make It Work? The Need for a Comprehensive Approach to Health and Welfare." *American Journal of Public Health* 9 (September 1982): 1028–33.

Starfield, Barbara H. et al. "Continuity and Coordination in Primary Care: Their Achievement and Utility." *Medical Care* 14 (July 1976): 625–36.

Vladeck, Bruce C. "Equity, Access and the Costs of Health Services." *Medical Care* 19 (December supplement 1981): 69–80.

Waldo, Daniel R. and Robert M. Gibson. "National Health Expenditures, 1981." *Health Care Financing Review* 4 (September 1982): 1–35.

Ware, John E. and Mary K. Snyder. "Dimensions of Patient Attitudes Regarding Doctors and Medical Care Services." *Medical Care* 13 (August 1975): 679–82.

Weiner, Stephen M. "Health Care Policy and Politics: Does the Past Tell Us Anything About the Future?" *American Journal of Law and Medicine* 5 (Winter 1980): 331–41.

Wilensky, Gail R. and Marc L. Berk. "Health Care, the Poor and the Role of Medicaid." *Health Affairs* (Fall 1982): 93–101.

Wolinsky, Fredric D. "Racial Differences in Illness Behavior." *Journal of Community Health* 8 (Winter 1982): 87–101.

Wolinsky, Fredric D. and William D. Marder. "Spending Time with Patients: The Impact of Organizational Structure on Medical Practice." *Medical Care* 20 (October 1982): 1051–1058.

Yergan, John et al. "Health Status as a Measure of Need for Medical Care: A Critique." *Medical Care* 19 (December 1981 supplement): 57–68.

# Appendix A *

## Sample Design, 1982 National Access Survey

### Selecting the sample

The universe for the 1982 National Access Survey was the U.S. population with home telephones. (A weight to adjust the data to approximate the total U.S. population is discussed toward the end of this appendix.) Because poor people generally have more medical care access problems, families whose 1981 income was less than 150 percent of the poverty level were oversampled. The family income cutoff levels used are shown in Table A.1.

---

*The principal author of this appendix was Martha J. Banks, CHAS Sampling Director.

Table A.1 Family Income Cutoffs — 150 Percent of Poverty Level

| Family Size | Income Cutoff |
|---|---|
| 1 | $ 7,200 |
| 2 | 9,200 |
| 3 | 10,900 |
| 4 | 14,000 |
| 5 | 16,500 |
| 6 | 18,700 |
| 7 | 21,100 |
| 8 | 23,500 |
| 9 plus | 28,000 |

The oversample of families below 150 percent of the poverty level was accomplished by creating two types of samples: a cross-sectional sample in which all contacted families were to be interviewed and a poverty sample in which only families below 150 percent of the poverty level were to be interviewed. Both of these types of samples were divided into half-samples so that the results of the first cross-section and the first poverty sample could be examined to see if the oversampling procedures should be adjusted before proceeding. Each cross-section sample was to yield 1500 interviews, while each oversample was to yield interviews with 900 families below 150 percent of the poverty level.

## The cross-section samples

Each cross-section was chosen from a frame of telephone numbers created by Survey Sampling, Inc. This frame consists of all listed and unlisted U.S. telephone numbers, in blocks (based on the last two digits of the phone numbers) containing three or more residential phone numbers out of 100 possible numbers. The phone numbers initially chosen formed an unclustered sample which was selected with probability inversely proportional to the number of residential phones per block of 100 numbers. If the initial sample phone number did not produce an interview (but rather a no answer after seven callbacks, a business, a refusal, etc.), it was replaced with another number from the same block. If this still did not result in an interview, the last two digits of the phone numbers were replaced with random numbers and the resulting number was assigned.

## The below 150 percent poverty oversamples

The phone numbers used in the oversamples were created by forming a specified number of phone numbers using the first eight digits of each of the phone numbers belonging to a cross-section family whose income was below 150 percent of the poverty level. About 315 clusters were associated with each half sample. Due to the geographic clustering of families below 150 percent of the poverty level and the geographic clustering of blocks of phone numbers, this procedure resulted in a set of clustered phone numbers with a higher-than-average chance of belonging to a family below 150 percent of the poverty level.

In the first oversample, phone numbers in each cluster were assigned until a fixed number of families had been screened for income. Overall the first oversample yielded interviews with about 1,100 poor and near-poor families. Only about 12 percent of them were Black (compared to the March 1982 Current Population Survey (CPS) estimate of 21 percent). A small part of the discrepancy in the two figures may be due to a possible differential phone coverage rate for poor Blacks and poor Whites. However, we believe the most likely explanation was differential response rates. It was decided that in the second oversample, clusters in which the associated cross-section poor or near-poor family was Black would be sampled at a higher rate than clusters in which the associated cross-section poor or near-poor family was White.

In each oversample, just as was true for the cross-sections, a total of eight calls was made to a number before the number was replaced by another number in the cluster.

## Sampling within families

Within each selected family, one adult and one child (if the family contained any children) were chosen for interview, with the adult most knowledgeable about the child's health responding for the child and the adult responding for himself or herself (with a few exceptions when this was not possible). The way in which the sample persons were chosen is shown on the first pages of the questionnaire (Appendix F). Each table had six variations, so that, overall, the persons selected within families reflect the proper mix of persons by age and sex.

### Number of completed interviews

Table A.2, based on Tables A-2 and A-3 of Harris (1982), presents the number of completed interviews by sample, age and poverty status.

## Weighting the data

Because of the oversampling of families below 150 percent of the poverty level, selection of one adult and one child within families, and for other reasons discussed below, the data from the 1982 National Access Survey must be weighted so that estimates can reflect the total U.S. population.

Table A.2 Number of Completed Interviews by
Type of Sample, Age and Poverty Status

| Sample | Total | Total Adults* | Children | Below 150% Poverty*** Total | Adults* | Children |
|---|---|---|---|---|---|---|
| Cross-sections | 4151** | 3014** | 1137 | 861 | 628 | 233 |
| First | 2075 | 1508 | 567 | 430 | 319 | 111 |
| Second | 2076** | 1506** | 570 | 431 | 309 | 122 |
| Oversamples | 2466 | 1795 | 671 | 2466 | 1795 | 671 |
| First | 1516 | 1104 | 412 | 1516 | 1104 | 412 |
| Second | 950 | 691 | 259 | 950 | 691 | 259 |
| Total | 6617** | 4809** | 1808 | 3327 | 2423 | 904 |

\*    This is also the number of families interviewed.
\*\*   Seven of these cases subsequently were removed because of the amount of missing information.
\*\*\* This sampling definition of the screening variable differs slightly from the analytic definition in that 235 persons in the cross-section were designated as below 150 percent of the poverty level through income imputation, while the answer to the income question of 17 oversample persons indicated they actually were above 150 percent of the poverty level.

## Weighting for selecting individuals within families

Because information was collected about one adult and child per family, individual-level data must be weighted by the number of adults or children in the family. For example, in a family consisting of two adults and three children, the interviewed adult would have a weight of 2 and the interviewed child would have a weight of 3.

The distribution of persons by this weight is shown in Table A.3.

Table A.3    Distribution of Weight Due to Selection of Individuals Within Families

| Weight | Number of Persons |
|---|---|
| 1 | 2189 |
| 2 | 3099 |
| 3 | 844 |
| 4 | 319 |
| 5 | 114 |
| 6 | 31 |
| 7 | 6 |
| 8 | 6 |
| 9 | 1 |
| 10 | 1 |

## Weighting for oversampling families below 150 percent of the poverty level

Because families below 150 percent of the poverty level were oversampled, the data must be weighted by a factor proportional to the inverse of the number of families interviewed per cluster. The distribution of interviewed persons and families by cluster size and the associated weight are given in Table A.4.

Table A.4    Distribution of Weight Due to the Oversampling of Families Below 150% of the Poverty Level

| Cluster Size | Number of Persons | Number of Families | Weight |
|---|---|---|---|
| 1 | 3180 | 2313 | 6.0 |
| 2 | 277 | 196 | 3.0 |
| 3 | 768 | 548 | 2.0 |
| 4 | 957 | 704 | 1.5 |
| 5 | 1418 | 1035 | 1.2 |
| 6 | 10 | 6 | 1.0 |

Weighting to reduce the nonphone noncoverage bias

Because the survey was conducted entirely by phone, only the U.S. population with telephones is represented by the data when weighted by the above weights. Even though most population groups have fairly high phone coverage, some groups with low coverage may have more severe access problems than the general population. To partially adjust for this bias, the data were weighted based on phone coverage rates obtained in the 1976 CHAS-NORC survey. These factors range from 1.000 to 1.982, with the categories being based on poverty status, age of head, race, region, residence, marital status of head and number of adults per family. The complete set of weights and further discussion are given in Banks (1983). The distribution of persons by this weight is shown in Table A.5.

### Table A.5 Distribution of Weight to Reduce the Nonphone Noncoverage Bias

| Weight | No. Persons | Weight | No. Persons | Weight | No. Persons |
|--------|-------------|--------|-------------|--------|-------------|
| 1.000 | 86 | 1.058 | 726 | 1.331 | 11 |
| 1.009 | 409 | 1.078 | 330 | 1.354 | 40 |
| 1.016 | 140 | 1.112 | 237 | 1.426 | 170 |
| 1.020 | 111 | 1.131 | 182 | 1.446 | 258 |
| 1.028 | 298 | 1.138 | 159 | 1.548 | 83 |
| 1.031 | 321 | 1.153 | 122 | 1.555 | 79 |
| 1.035 | 279 | 1.162 | 341 | 1.600 | 86 |
| 1.038 | 439 | 1.164 | 309 | 1.881 | 130 |
| 1.045 | 453 | 1.219 | 74 | 1.947 | 16 |
| 1.046 | 272 | 1.251 | 180 | 1.982 | 81 |
| 1.054 | 188 | | | | |

## Post-stratification weighting

The process of applying a set of weights that adjusts the sample distribution according to the distribution obtained in more reliable data is known as post-stratification. The 1982 National Access data set was adjusted using information from the March 1982 Current Population Survey (CPS). In the CPS, information was collected on all persons in about 59,000 households representing the U.S. population. Therefore, these estimates can be expected to be more reliable than estimates based on data for one or two persons in 4,800 families. Additionally, two problems caused the post-stratification weights to be more variable than expected: a low response rate* and the handling of multifamily households. They make post-stratification absolutely necessary when analyzing the data. Unfortunately, post-stratification only partially corrects for the problems. The post-stratification weights used are

Table A.6 Distribution of Post-stratification Weights

Race and Poverty Status

| Age and Family Size | Black | | | Other | | |
|---|---|---|---|---|---|---|
| | Below Poverty | 100%- 150% Poverty | 150% Plus Poverty | Below Poverty | 100%- 150% Poverty | 150% Plus Poverty |
| 0–17 | .5617 | .3880 | .5047 | .3959 | .3366 | .3993 |
| 18–64 1 | 1.2037 | .5643 | .5654 | 1.2037 | .5643 | .5654 |
| 18–64 2+ | .4920 | .3561 | .5991 | .3242 | .2380 | .4088 |
| 65+ 1 | .5499 | .5499 | .7385 | .4402 | .4895 | .7385 |
| 65+ 2+ | .5499 | .5499 | .7833 | .1449 | .2084 | .7833 |

*CHAS estimated the response rates for the cross-section and oversamples to be 60.8 percent and 58.9 percent, respectively.

given in Table A.6. The CPS distribution used in this adjustment is given in Table 7 of U.S. Bureau of the Census (1983). Once all weights are applied, the estimate in each of the 30 cells will equal one ten-thousandth of the U.S. population estimate.

Table A.7 Distribution of Overall Weights for Individuals

| Overall Individual Weight | Total | Poverty Status | | |
|---|---|---|---|---|
| | | Below Poverty | 100% to 150% Poverty | 150% Plus Poverty |
| 0.30– 0.50 | 187 | 71 | 116 | 0 |
| 0.50– 0.75 | 787 | 226 | 556 | 5 |
| 0.75– 1.00 | 656 | 196 | 447 | 13 |
| 1.00– 1.50 | 715 | 265 | 417 | 33 |
| 1.50– 2.00 | 420 | 212 | 173 | 35 |
| 2.00– 2.50 | 522 | 155 | 101 | 266 |
| 2.50– 3.00 | 353 | 140 | 50 | 163 |
| 3.00– 3.50 | 231 | 63 | 60 | 108 |
| 3.50– 4.00 | 294 | 41 | 20 | 233 |
| 4.00– 4.50 | 52 | 31 | 10 | 11 |
| 4.50– 5.00 | 528 | 31 | 15 | 482 |
| 5.00– 5.50 | 734 | 10 | 1 | 723 |
| 5.50– 6.00 | 241 | 17 | 0 | 224 |
| 6.00– 7.00 | 62 | 14 | 6 | 42 |
| 7.00– 8.00 | 401 | 11 | 3 | 387 |
| 8.00– 9.00 | 49 | 7 | 2 | 40 |
| 9.00–10.00 | 180 | 6 | 2 | 172 |
| 10.00–12.50 | 96 | 10 | 1 | 85 |
| 12.50–15.00 | 102 | 14 | 2 | 86 |
| Median | 2.565 | 1.500 | .928 | 5.141 |
| Mean | 3.437 | 2.083 | 1.226 | 5.509 |

## Overall weight distribution

A summary of the overall weight distribution for individuals is given in Table A.7. The overall weight is computed by multiplying together each of the four weights discussed above. (There were some exceptions to this, due to the presence of some extremely large weights. All weights above 15 were lowered to 15, and weights between 10 and 15 were raised slightly to compensate.) When a family-level file is used, the within-family individual weight component is not used. The overall family weight has a mean value of 2.471.

# References

Banks, Martha J. "Comparing Health and Medical Care Estimates of the Phone and Nonphone Populations." In *Proceedings of the American Statistical Association Section on Survey Research Methods.* Washington, DC: American Statistical Association. 1983.

Louis Harris and Associates, Inc. *Access to Health Care Services in the United States: 1982.* New York: Louis Harris and Associates, Inc. 1982.

U.S. Bureau of the Census. *Money Income and Poverty Status of Families and Persons in the United States: 1981 (Final Report from the March 1982 Current Population Survey).* Series P-60, #144. Washington, DC: Government Printing Office. 1983.

# Appendix B *

## Standard Errors of Estimates, 1982 National Access Survey

### General discussion of standard errors

The particular sample chosen for the 1982 National Access Study was one of a large number of possible samples of the same size that could have been selected using the sample design. Estimates derived from any of these samples would differ from those derived from the others. The deviation of a sample estimate from the average of all possible samples is called the sampling error. The standard error of a survey estimate is a measure of the variation among the estimates from the possible samples; thus it measures the precision with which an estimate from a particular sample approximates the average result of all possible samples.

---

*The principal author of this appendix was Martha J. Banks, CHAS Sampling Director.

As calculated for this report, the standard error also partially measures the effect of nonsampling errors but does not measure any systematic biases in the data. Bias is the difference, averaged over all possible samples, between the estimate and the desired value. Obviously, the accuracy of a survey result depends upon both the sampling and nonsampling error measured by the standard error, and the bias and other types of nonsampling error not measured by the standard error.

The sample estimate and an estimate of its standard error permit us to construct interval estimates with prescribed levels of confidence so that the interval includes the average result of all possible samples. To illustrate, if all possible samples were selected, each of these were surveyed under essentially the same conditions, and an estimate and its estimated standard error were calculated for each sample, then:

1. Approximately two-thirds of the interval from one standard error below the estimate to one standard error above the estimate would include the average value of all possible samples. We call an interval from one standard error below the estimate to one standard error above the estimate a 68 percent confidence interval.

2. Approximately nine-tenths of the interval from 1.6 standard errors below the estimate to 1.6 standard errors above the estimate would include the average value of all possible samples. We call an interval from 1.6 standard errors below the estimate to 1.6 standard errors above the estimate a 90 percent confidence interval.

3. Approximately nineteen-twentieths of the interval from two standard errors below the estimate to two standard errors above the estimate would include the average value of all possible samples. We call an interval from two standard errors below the estimate to two standard errors above the estimate a 95 percent confidence interval.

4. Almost all intervals from three standard errors below the sample estimate to three standard errors above the sample estimate would include the average value of all possible samples.

Thus for a *particular* sample, one can say with specified confidence that the average of all possible samples is included in the constructed interval.

For simplicity's sake, we will use only the 68 percent and the 95 percent confidence intervals in further discussion. In the text, the 95 percent confidence interval was applied most often.

*Cautionary remark:* The 68 percent confidence interval will exclude the expected value (the average value of all possible samples) 32 percent of the time, on the average. Similarly, the 95 percent confidence interval will exclude the expected value 5 percent of the time. Thus, when examining a number of estimates, one out of 20 can be expected to appear at the 95 percent confidence level to be different from a hypothesized value, even though none of them actually are different. Consequently, in order to avoid any inference that sample results are significant when they are not, traditional statistical theory demands that hypotheses be made before the data is examined. Not doing so increases the likelihood of accepting false hypotheses. Goodman (1969) discusses a method which avoids this problem by applying factors to individual estimates of the standard errors.

## Standard error estimates, 1982 National Access Survey

Standard errors for estimates from complex surveys traditionally are calculated by computing simple random sample standard errors and multiplying by a factor which takes the design complexities into account. These factors are called design factors and were obtained by computing standard errors for a sample of estimates in this report and generalizing the results. Thus they provide an indication of the size of the standard error rather than the precise standard error for any specific item.

Design factors can be obtained by identifying the appropriate category in Table B.1 and using the corresponding estimate for the design factor. Table B.2 contains the categories applicable to the major access variables used in the analyses. Tables B.3 and B.4 give the number of interviewed persons and families, respectively, that were the basis for the major estimates in this report.

## Standard errors of percents

To calculate the standard error of a percent, multiply the percent by 100 minus the percent, divide by the unweighted number of cases represented in the denominator of the percent, take the square root and multiply by the appropriate design factor.

*Illustration.* Table 2.1 indicates that about 17 percent of all persons 18 to 34 years old had no regular source of care in 1982. The correlation of age and source of care between families within a cluster is low (the within-family correlation is immaterial, because only one person per age group was interviewed), so we use a design factor from Table B.1 of 1.35. Table B.3 indicates that the 1982 estimates are based on 1798 persons 18 to 34. The standard error of the 17 percent estimated persons 18 to 34 who had no regular source of care is 1.35 SQRT [ (17)(83)/(1798) ] = 1.20. Two standard errors is 2.39 which rounds to 2, so we can conclude with 95 percent confidence that the average estimate from all possible samples would be between 15 percent and 19 percent $(17 - 2, 17 + 2)$. We can conclude with 68 percent confidence that the average estimate would be between 16 percent and 18 percent.

## Standard errors of means

The sampling variability of an estimated mean depends on the form of the distribution as well as on the number of sample cases. Estimated standard errors of means appearing in this report were calculated by multiplying the design factor by the standard error calculated for a simple random sample having this sample's weighted distribution and unweighted number of cases. Text tables containing means also contain standard error estimates of these means.

## Standard errors of ratios

The standard error ($\sigma$) of a ratio (A/B) can be obtained from the formula:

$$\sigma_{A/B} = A/B \; SQRT \; [(\sigma_A/A)^2 + (\sigma_B/B)^2 - 2\rho\sigma_A\sigma_B/AB].$$

The values for $\rho$, the correlation between A and B, were estimated to be .9 for the ratio of emergency room and outpatient department use to total ambulatory use.

## Standard errors of differences

For a difference between two sample estimates (A and B), the standard error is obtained from the formula:

$$\sigma_{A-B} = SQRT \; (\sigma_A^2 + \sigma_B^2 - 2\rho\sigma_A\sigma_B)$$

where $\rho$ is the correlation between A and B. When B is a subclass of A, $\rho = \sigma_A/\sigma_B$. Otherwise, using a value of zero for $\rho$ usually will result in only a slight overestimate of the standard error of the difference.

*Illustration.* We have calculated that the estimated 17 percent of all persons 18 to 34 years old had no regular source of care in 1982. For the nation as a whole, the estimate is 11 percent, and the standard error is 1.45 SQRT [(11) (89)/6610] = .056. A design factor of 1.45 is used because the within-family correlation is medium and the between-family correlation is low.

The standard error of the apparent 6 percent difference between all persons and those 18 to 34 years old is

SQRT $[(1.20)^2 + (0.56)^2 - 2(0.56/1.20)\ (1.20)\ (0.56)] = 1.06$

The 95 percent confidence interval ranges from $6 - 2 = 4$ percent to $6 + 2 = 8$ percent. Therefore it can be said with 95 percent confidence that a larger percent of persons 18 to 34 have no regular source of care than is true for persons of all ages.

## Standard error estimates, other data sources

Standard error estimates based on other data sources are used in a manner similar to that described above. For 1976 estimates appearing in this report, design factors are 3.64 for Hispanics, 2.02 for nonwhites, and 1.35 for other estimates. In all, 7,787 persons were interviewed. (For further information consult Appendix B in Aday, et al., 1980.) Standard errors for 1970 and other prior years can be found in Andersen, et al., 1976, Appendix I. Those for NCHS data appear in NCHS, 1982.

## References

Aday, Lu Ann et al. *Health Care in the U.S.: Equitable for Whom?* Beverly Hills, CA: Sage Publications. 1980.

Andersen, Ronald et al. *Two Decades of Health Services: Social Survey Trends in Use and Expenditures*. Cambridge, MA: Ballinger. 1976.

Goodman, Leo A. "Ransacking Cross-Classification Tables." *American Journal of Sociology* 75 (July 1969): 1–40.

NCHS (National Center for Health Statistics). *Current Estimates from the National Health Interview Survey: United States, 1981*. DHHS Publication No. (PHS) 82-1569. Washington, DC: Government Printing Office. 1982.

# TABLE B.1 Design Factors for Various Categories of Estimates: 1982

|  | CATEGORIES OF ESTIMATES | | | |
|---|---|---|---|---|
|  |  | Correlation | | |
| Universe (a) | Within Family | Between Family Within Cluster | Independent or Dependent Variable (b) | Design Factors |
| all persons | high | high | any age group | 1.59 |
| all persons | high | high | below 1.5 poverty | 3.14 |
| all persons | high | high | 1.5 poverty and above | 1.28 |
| all persons | high | high | other than above 3 categories | 1.84 |
| all persons | high | medium | any age group | 1.46 |
| all persons | high | medium | below 1.5 poverty | 2.44 |
| all persons | high | medium | 1.5 poverty and above | 1.28 |
| all persons | high | medium | other than above 3 categories | 1.69 |
| all persons | high | low | any age group | 1.35 |
| all persons | high | low | below 1.5 poverty | 1.90 |
| all persons | high | low | 1.5 poverty and above | 1.28 |
| all persons | high | low | other than above 3 categories | 1.56 |
| all persons | medium | medium | any age group | 1.46 |
| all persons | medium | medium | below 1.5 poverty and above | 2.26 |
| all persons | medium | medium | 1.5 poverty and above | 1.19 |
| all persons | medium | medium | other than above 3 categories | 1.56 |
| all persons | medium | low | any age group | 1.35 |
| all persons | medium | low | below 1.5 poverty | 1.76 |
| all persons | medium | low | 1.5 poverty and above | 1.19 |
| all persons | medium | low | other than above 3 categories | 1.45 |
| all persons | low | low | any age group | 1.35 |
| all persons | low | low | below 1.5 poverty | 1.68 |
| all persons | low | low | 1.5 poverty and above | 1.13 |
| all persons | low | low | other than above 3 categories | 1.38 |

(a) The categories of estimates and design factors noted for "adults only" apply to estimates applicable to "children only" as well.

(b) Also included in the "below 1.5 poverty" and "1.5 poverty and above" categories are any subclasses of the variable. For instance for "below 1.5 poverty" this would include the below poverty population and the Medicaid population. The "1.5 poverty and above" includes high income people.

**TABLE B.1 (continued)  Design Factors for Various Categories of Estimates: 1982**

CATEGORIES OF ESTIMATES

| Universe (a) | Correlation Within Family | Between Family, Within Cluster | Independent or Dependent Variable (b) | Design Factors |
|---|---|---|---|---|
| adults only | NA | high | any age group | 1.59 |
| adults only | NA | high | below 1.5 poverty | 2.71 |
| adults only | NA | high | 1.5 poverty and above | 1.11 |
| adults only | NA | high | other than above 3 categories | 1.59 |
| adults only | NA | medium | any age group | 1.46 |
| adults only | NA | medium | below 1.5 poverty | 2.11 |
| adults only | NA | medium | 1.5 poverty and above | 1.11 |
| adults only | NA | medium | other than above 3 categories | 1.46 |
| adults only | NA | low | any age group | 1.35 |
| adults only | NA | low | below 1.5 poverty | 1.64 |
| adults only | NA | low | 1.5 poverty and above | 1.11 |
| adults only | NA | low | other than above 3 categories | 1.35 |
| families | NA | high | any age group | 1.50 |
| families | NA | high | below 1.5 poverty and above | 2.51 |
| families | NA | high | 1.5 poverty and above | 1.05 |
| families | NA | high | other than above 3 categories | 2.30 |
| families | NA | medium | any age group | 1.38 |
| families | NA | medium | below 1.5 poverty | 1.95 |
| families | NA | medium | 1.5 poverty and above | 1.05 |
| families | NA | medium | other than above 3 categories | 1.79 |
| families | NA | low | any age group | 1.27 |
| families | NA | low | below 1.5 poverty | 1.52 |
| families | NA | low | 1.5 poverty and above | 1.05 |
| families | NA | low | Other than above 3 categories | 1.40 |

(a) The categories of estimates and design factors noted for "adults only" apply to estimates applicable to "children only" as well.

(b) Also included in the "below 1.5 poverty" and "1.5 poverty and above" categories are any subclasses of the variable. For instance for "below 1.5 poverty" this would include the below poverty population and the Medicaid population. The "1.5 poverty and above" includes high income people.

# TABLE B.2 Classification of Major Access Variables by Categories of Estimates: 1982

| MAJOR ACCESS VARIABLES (a) | Universe | CATEGORIES OF ESTIMATES (b) Correlation | |
|---|---|---|---|
| | | Within Family | Between Family, Within Cluster |
| DIFFICULT TO GET MEDICAL HELP | families | NA | low |
| HOSPITALIZATION | all persons | low | low |
| ILLNESS, SERIOUSLY ILL FAMILY MEMBER | families | NA | low |
| INCOME, REDUCED DUE TO ILLNESS | families | NA | low |
| INSURANCE COVERAGE | all persons | high | medium |
| INSURANCE COVERAGE, CHANGES IN | adults only | NA | low |
| MEDICAL EMERGENCY | all persons | low | low |
| NEEDED CARE BUT DID NOT GET IT | families | NA | low |
| NEEDED SPECIAL SERVICES BUT DID NOT GET THEM | families | NA | low |
| OFFICE WAITING TIME, RECENT MEDICAL VISIT | all persons | medium | low |
| PHYSICIAN VISITS | all persons | low | low |
| PREVENTIVE CARE | adults only | NA | low |
| | children only | NA | medium |
| REFUSED CARE FOR FINANCIAL REASONS | families | NA | low |
| REGULAR SOURCE, LOCATION | all persons | medium | low |
| REGULAR SOURCE, TYPE OF | all persons | medium | low |
| SATISFACTION WITH RECENT VISIT | all persons | low | low |
| TROUBLE, FAMILIES IN | families | NA | low |
| WOULD GO SOURCE, LOCATION | all persons | medium | low |

(a) See Appendix C for definition of variables.

(b) See Table B.1 for design factors associated with respective categories of estimates.

## TABLE B.3 Unweighted Number of Sample Persons for Major Analytic Subgroups by Selected Population Subgroups: 1982

| SELECTED POPULATION SUBGROUPS | TOTAL PERSONS | AGE 0-16 | AGE AND 17+ | 17+ FEMALE | HAVE A REGULAR SOURCE OF CARE | SAW PHYSICIAN IN THE YEAR | RECENT VISIT. REPORTED ON Satisfaction | Waiting Time | HOSPITALIZED IN THE YEAR | MEDICAL EMERGENCY IN THE YEAR | ADULTS WHOSE INSURANCE COVERAGE CHANGED Total | Less |
|---|---|---|---|---|---|---|---|---|---|---|---|---|
| **AGE** | | | | | | | | | | | | |
| Infants | 56 | 56 | – | – | 55 | 56 | 56 | – | 0 | 6 | – | – |
| 1-5 | 584 | 584 | – | – | 556 | 543 | 552 | – | 53 | 122 | – | – |
| 6-17 | 1252 | 1148 | 100 | 54 | 1151 | 962 | 859 | 64 | 52 | 178 | 3 | 1 |
| 18-34 | 1798 | – | 1798 | 981 | 1464 | 1472 | 1312 | 1312 | 237 | 272 | 346 | 104 |
| 35-54 | 1206 | – | 1206 | 612 | 1050 | 915 | 815 | 815 | 122 | 170 | 258 | 76 |
| 55-64 | 668 | – | 668 | 381 | 606 | 535 | 469 | 469 | 90 | 95 | 115 | 44 |
| 65+ | 1046 | – | 1046 | 666 | 961 | 900 | 771 | 771 | 208 | 136 | 148 | 28 |
| **RESIDENCE** | | | | | | | | | | | | |
| **SMSA** | | | | | | | | | | | | |
| Central City | 1945 | 492 | 1386 | 847 | 1690 | 1596 | 1433 | 1050 | 213 | 300 | 237 | 70 |
| Other | 2870 | 809 | 1921 | 1103 | 2543 | 2365 | 2045 | 1479 | 312 | 439 | 392 | 105 |
| **Non SMSA** | | | | | | | | | | | | |
| Non Farm | 1482 | 391 | 1044 | 630 | 1336 | 1194 | 1018 | 762 | 202 | 201 | 211 | 69 |
| Farm | 302 | 87 | 197 | 114 | 274 | 228 | 196 | 140 | 35 | 39 | 30 | 9 |
| **FAMILY INCOME** | | | | | | | | | | | | |
| Low | 3913 | 943 | 2780 | 1825 | 3421 | 3168 | 2726 | 2085 | 530 | 595 | 452 | 147 |
| Medium | 1124 | 348 | 747 | 378 | 983 | 893 | 801 | 544 | 100 | 160 | 159 | 39 |
| High | 1573 | 488 | 1021 | 491 | 1439 | 1322 | 1165 | 802 | 132 | 224 | 259 | 67 |
| **ETHNICITY** | | | | | | | | | | | | |
| Hispanic | 563 | 194 | 344 | 190 | 479 | 448 | 392 | 265 | 48 | 88 | 67 | 24 |
| Non Hispanic White | 5264 | 1343 | 3695 | 2179 | 4679 | 4291 | 3750 | 2784 | 643 | 775 | 735 | 199 |
| Black | 688 | 211 | 448 | 289 | 605 | 569 | 486 | 340 | 63 | 104 | 61 | 27 |
| **150% POVERTY LEVEL BY RACE** | | | | | | | | | | | | |
| **Poor** | | | | | | | | | | | | |
| White | 2895 | 723 | 2025 | 1338 | 2543 | 2328 | 2001 | 1520 | 415 | 436 | 332 | 107 |
| Nonwhite | 607 | 194 | 385 | 260 | 535 | 497 | 420 | 290 | 65 | 97 | 41 | 25 |
| **Non Poor** | | | | | | | | | | | | |
| White | 2845 | 778 | 1967 | 1000 | 2543 | 2343 | 2083 | 1490 | 269 | 412 | 464 | 112 |
| Nonwhite | 263 | 84 | 171 | 96 | 222 | 215 | 188 | 131 | 13 | 34 | 33 | 9 |
| **MAIN EARNER EMPLOYMENT STATUS** | | | | | | | | | | | | |
| Employed | 4528 | 1436 | 2942 | 1615 | 3988 | 3636 | 3228 | 2166 | 412 | 650 | 608 | 161 |
| Not employed | 460 | 173 | 271 | 160 | 386 | 365 | 322 | 194 | 45 | 73 | 54 | 28 |
| Not in labor force | 1577 | 156 | 1308 | 903 | 1435 | 1347 | 1112 | 1050 | 299 | 246 | 205 | 62 |
| **INSURANCE COVERAGE** | | | | | | | | | | | | |
| Private only | 4027 | 1275 | 2630 | 1423 | 3609 | 3292 | 2940 | 1980 | 375 | 363 | 573 | 140 |
| Public only | 466 | 76 | 358 | 259 | 425 | 410 | 351 | 301 | 88 | 66 | 65 | 26 |
| Public and private | 845 | 97 | 685 | 445 | 784 | 731 | 595 | 560 | 167 | 121 | 133 | 29 |
| No insurance | 703 | 217 | 461 | 275 | 528 | 486 | 423 | 275 | 48 | 66 | 40 | 36 |
| **TOTAL** | 6610 | 1788 | 4548 | 2694 | 5843 | 5383 | 4692 | 3431 | 762 | 979 | 870 | 253 |

**TABLE B.4 Unweighted Number of Families for Major Analytic Subgroups by Selected Population Subgroups: 1982**

| SELECTED POPULATION SUBGROUPS | TOTAL FAMILIES | MAJOR ANALYTIC SUBGROUPS | | |
|---|---|---|---|---|
| | | EARNINGS REDUCED DUE TO ILLNESS | NEEDED CARE BUT DID NOT GET | SERIOUSLY ILL FAMILY MEMBER |
| RESIDENCE | | | | |
| SMSA | | | | |
| Central City | 1413 | 98 | 99 | 153 |
| Other | 1986 | 122 | 138 | 221 |
| Non SMSA | | | | |
| Non Farm | 1074 | 70 | 71 | 111 |
| Farm | 204 | 9 | 13 | 21 |
| FAMILY INCOME | | | | |
| Low | 2864 | 214 | 247 | 359 |
| Medium | 755 | 50 | 33 | 59 |
| High | 1058 | 35 | 41 | 88 |
| ETHNICITY | | | | |
| Hispanic | 362 | 27 | 33 | 45 |
| Non Hispanic | | | | |
| White | 3800 | 240 | 240 | 409 |
| Black | 453 | 30 | 41 | 47 |
| 150% POVERTY LEVEL | | | | |
| BY RACE | | | | |
| Poor | | | | |
| White | 2113 | 178 | 183 | 274 |
| Nonwhite | 389 | 28 | 43 | 45 |
| Non Poor | | | | |
| White | 2000 | 175 | 86 | 86 |
| Nonwhite | 175 | 7 | 9 | 12 |
| MAIN EARNER | | | | |
| EMPLOYMENT STATUS | | | | |
| Employed | 3006 | 184 | 215 | 243 |
| Not employed | 278 | 20 | 29 | 32 |
| Not in labor force | 1371 | 91 | 77 | 226 |
| INSURANCE COVERAGE | | | | |
| Private only | 2676 | 170 | 151 | 234 |
| Public only | 376 | 25 | 29 | 65 |
| Public and private | 728 | 38 | 39 | 111 |
| No insurance | 469 | 43 | 75 | 48 |
| TOTAL | 4677 | 299 | 321 | 506 |

# Appendix C
## Definition of Variables

### Age

Age refers to age at the actual date of the interview. Any missing age values were imputed based on the family composition and other characteristics of the respondent.

### Difficult to get medical help

Respondents were asked, "In the last 12 months, has it been easier or more difficult for you and your family to get the medical help you need, or hasn't it changed in the last year?" Responses were "easier," "more difficult" or "hasn't changed."

### Disability days

Disability days includes estimates of bed days and other days in which respondents may have had to cut down on the things they usually do. Bed days refers to the number of days respondents had to stay in bed in the year, based on the question, "How many days *altogether* during the past year, that is, since (*Date one year ago*) 1981, did you stay in bed more than half of the day because of illness or injury?" Days spent overnight in a hospital are excluded from the bed days estimates reported here. In addition to the question to elicit bed days, respondents were asked, "*Not counting the days in bed,* how many days during the past year, that is, since (*Date one year ago*) 1981, did you have to *cut down* on the things you usually do for more than half of the day because of illness or injury?" Bed days (excluding hospital days) and other restricted activity days were summed to obtain the *total* disability days.

## Education, main wage earner

Respondents were asked, "What was the last grade of school that the main wage earner completed?" Categories included no formal schooling, first through seventh grade, eighth grade, some high school, high school graduate, some college, two-year college graduate, four-year college graduate, postgraduate or trade/technical/vocational after high school.

## Employment status, main wage earner

Respondents were asked, "Which of the following *best* describes (his/her) current employment situation?" The response categories provided were: working full-time, working part-time, laid off or on strike, unemployed (looking for work), unemployed (not looking for work), retired, unable to work (disabled), keeping house or full-time student. The main wage earner's employment status was assigned to the sampled adult and child record in the family and is the employment status reported in the tables. [See Aday, et al. (1980: 280) for questions used in 1970 and 1976.]

## Ethnicity

Ethnicity was elicited by the question, "Are you of Hispanic origin or not?" and, "Do you consider yourself White, Black, Oriental or what?" Those who said "yes" to the Hispanic origin question were assigned this status, regardless of their racial classification. All non-Hispanics were then assigned to the White, Black or other (Oriental and other race) categories, based on their response to the racial classification question. In the 1970 and 1976 studies Hispanics are not identified, but are included in the White or Black groups as appropriate.

## Family size

Family size was based on the total number of adults and children related by blood, marriage or adoption living in the family unit.

## Hospitalization

*Hospitalized in the year.* Respondents were asked, "Have you been a patient overnight in a hospital during the past 12 months, since (*Date one year ago*) 1981?" [See Aday, et al. (1980: 281) for 1976 item.]

*Hospital admissions.* For those who were hospitalized, the number of admissions was obtained by asking, "How many times were you admitted to hospital since (*Date one year ago*) 1981?"

*Hospital nights.* Nights hospitalized were elicited by asking, "Altogether, how many nights did you stay in a hospital during that period, that is since (*Date one year ago*) 1981?"

## Illness, seriously ill family member

Adult respondents were asked whether any family member living in the household has a serious illness, is chronically sick or needs medical treatment or hospitalization on a regular basis. Respondents who answered "yes" were then asked to identify the family members and their illnesses or conditions, if the family member(s) need to have someone present in the house at all times, if anyone in the family made a major change in job, housing or living arrangements because of that person's illness and the nature of that change.

Respondents with serious or chronically ill family members were also asked if they had looked for but were unable to obtain the following services: home visits from a physical therapist, mental health counselor or social worker, or nurse; a housekeeper; meals on wheels; transportation to the doctor or hospital; medical applicances or equipment for home use; home dental care, or nursing home or any other long-term care outside of the home. The last question for these respondents was, "How serious a *financial* problem has illness been to your family in the last year—has it been a major problem, a minor problem or no financial problem at all?"

## Income, total family

The designations of low, middle and high family income categories for the 1963, 1970 and 1976 CHAS-NORC surveys and the 1982 National Access Survey were altered in each study to adjust for inflation estimates published by the U.S. Bureau of Labor Statistics. The income cutting points for each study are summarized in Table C.1.

Table C.1 Total Family Income Cutting Points

| | Low | Income Categories<br>Medium | High |
|---|---|---|---|
| 1963 | LE $ 3,999 | $ 4,000– 6,999 | $ 7,000 + |
| 1970 | LE 5,999 | 6,000–10,999 | 11,000 + |
| 1976 | LE 7,999 | 8,000–14,999 | 15,000 + |
| 1982 | LE 15,000 | 15,001–25,000 | 25,001 + |

## Income, poverty level

The poverty level cutoffs were based on a poverty index developed by the Social Security Administration, which provides a range of cutoffs adjusted by family size, sex of the family head and farm or nonfarm residence. At the core of this definition of poverty was a nutritionally adequate food plan designed by the Department of Agriculture. The cutoff points were based on a table of "Poverty Cutoffs" for 1975, published in *Current Population Reports*, Series P-60, no. 103. The levels provided in Table 16 of that report were multiplied by 1.25 to include more of the marginal poor in the "poverty level" category. The resulting cutting points adjusted for inflation (CPI) for subsequent years are shown in Table C.2. Families were considered to be below the poverty level if they reported their annual income to be less than or equal to the specified amounts. In the 1982 National Access Study, the poverty level cutoffs were based on *family size only*, multiplied by 1.50 (150 percent of poverty level). Because different cutoffs were used in 1976 and 1982, comparisons by poverty level over time are not emphasized.

## Table C.2 Poverty Level Cutting Points
### CHAS-NORC, 1976

| Size of Family | Nonfarm | | Farm | |
|---|---|---|---|---|
| | Male Head | Female Head | Male Head | Female Head |
| 1 | $ 3,564 | $ 3,294 | $ 2,995 | $ 2,780 |
| 2 | 4,394 | 4,325 | 3,704 | 3,543 |
| 3 | 5,396 | 5,219 | 4,565 | 4,350 |
| 4 | 6,878 | 6,841 | 5,871 | 4,616 |
| 5 | 8,130 | 8,043 | 6,940 | 6,994 |
| 6 | 9,153 | 9,088 | 7,788 | 7,631 |
| 7 or more | 11,320 | 11,023 | 9,549 | 9,559 |

### National Access Survey, 1982

| | |
|---|---|
| 1 | $ 7,200 |
| 2 | 9,200 |
| 3 | 10,900 |
| 4 | 14,000 |
| 5 | 16,500 |
| 6 | 18,700 |
| 7 | 21,100 |
| 8 | 23,500 |
| 9 or more | 28,000 |

## Income, Reduced Due To Illness

Families were asked, "In the last year have the earnings of your family been reduced by a health problem or disability of a wage earner or not?" A family who responded that the family earnings had been reduced was then asked, "Has the income of your family been seriously reduced, reduced somewhat or reduced a little because of the illness of a wage earner?"

## Insurance Coverage

A person is said to have group coverage if he or she reports that health insurance is provided through place of work or other group membership (Grange, Farm Bureau, Medical Society, group retirement plan and so on). Persons who said they bought their health insurance directly were reported to have "individual" coverage. Respondents were characterized as having Medicaid or reduced price care if they were covered by Medicaid, Public Aid or other health care center where they could get care at no cost or reduced rates.

The private and public insurance coverage status for persons of all ages (including persons under 65) refer, respectively, to whether they have group coverage through work or union, an individually-purchased policy or both, or Medicaid, Medicare or both, or if they don't have *any* form of public, private or other (e.g. VA, workmen's compensation, etc.) coverage, i.e., are uninsured.

In the 1982 study *only* adult respondents were asked about insurance coverage. This information was used to provide insurance coverage estimates for the U.S. adult population. Estimates for the total U.S. population were derived by assigning, within each family, the adult respondent's coverage to the child respondent. If the adult respondent had Medicare coverage, however, the child was assigned "other" coverage status. The same approach was used with the 1976 data to enhance comparability.

## Insurance coverage, changes in

Adult respondents were asked, "Has your health coverage, that is, the benefits provided by your health insurance, changed in the last year since *(Date one year ago)* 1981, or not?" If there had been a change, respondents were asked *how* (price of policy changed, coverage dropped or reduced or increased, or changed insurer) and *why* (changed or lost job, etc.), and if, as a result of the change, the respondent had been unable to get some kind of health care, changed his or her regular source of care or put off getting care.

## Insurance coverage, type of

Persons who reported they had health insurance were asked to indicate which of the following kinds of coverage their plan(s) provided: hospital expenses, surgical expenses, charges for prescribed medicine taken outside the hospital or charges for visits to a doctor's office.

Table C.3 summarizes an estimation matrix used to assign coverage to individuals who did not report having coverage under the respective plans. For 1976, coverage was assigned as basically "yes" or "no." For 1982, coverage was assigned as "all" or "some."

## Length of time in community

Respondents were asked, "For how many years have you lived in this community?"

## Medical emergency

If a respondent had a medical emergency any time in the last year, he or she was asked where he or she went for emergency care, the condition which caused the emergency, if he or she had problems getting there what these problems were, and if he or she was completely, somewhat or not at all satisfied with various aspects of the care.

The places for emergency care were: doctor's office or private clinic; company or union clinic; school or unspecified clinic; neighborhood or government-sponsored

Table C.3 Types of Insurance which People Were Estimated to Have, Based on Coverage

| | Hospital | | | Surgical | | | Outpatient Drugs | | | Outpatient Physician Visits | | |
|---|---|---|---|---|---|---|---|---|---|---|---|---|
| | 1976 Yes | 1982 All | Some | 1976 Yes | 1982 All | Some | 1976 Yes | 1982 All | Some | 1976 Yes | 1982 All | Some |
| Medicare, Part A | X | | X | | | | | | | | | |
| Medicare, Part B | | | | X | | X | | | | X | | X |
| Medicaid | X | X | | X | X | | X | | X | X | X | |
| Clinic with reduced rates | | | | | | | | | | X | | X |

159

clinic, hospital outpatient clinic or unspecified hospital clinic; hospital emergency room; health maintenance organization; or other location.

Satisfaction was asked about: the amount of time to get there; the amount of time waiting to see the doctor; the amount of time the doctor spent with the person; the information given to the person about what was wrong or what was being done; the out-of-pocket cost; the quality of care; and the overall visit. Response categories provided were completely, somewhat or not at all satisfied.

## Needed care but did not get it

Adult respondents were asked, "The next questions apply to you and all other members of your family *who live with you*. Was there any time in the last year--since *(Date one year ago)* 1981--that you felt you or a member of your family living with you needed medical help but did not get it for some reason?"

Respondents answering "yes" were asked which family members needed help but didn't get it, and which one had the most recent episode. Then, the respondents were asked, "Thinking about the most recent time this happened, did *anyone in your family try* to get medical help?" If a family member tried to get help, the respondent was asked the main reason that his or her family was not able to get the medical help needed in this situation. If a family member did not try to get help, the respondent was asked, "What was the *main* reason no one in your family tried to see a doctor about this situation?" The response categories provided were as follows:

a)  could not get an appointment,
b)  did not know a good doctor or clinic to go to,
c)  it cost too much,
d)  could not get off work,

e) couldn't find anyone to take care of the children,
f) would have had to wait too long in the doctor's office or clinic,
g) there was no easy way to get to the doctor's office or clinic,
h) couldn't find a doctor who speaks your language,
i) not covered by insurance,
j) too nervous or afraid or
k) other reason.

## Needed special services but did not get them

Families who needed, but did not obtain, special health care services for any reason are those in which at least one family member did not get any one of the following: a) emergency medical care, b) overnight hospital stay, c) services at home, such as visiting nurse or doctor, d) mental health services or psychiatric counseling, e) treatment of drug or drinking problem, f) family planning services or birth control, g) services of a pharmacy or drugstore at night or on weekends, h) nursing home facilities, i) services of a pediatrician or children's doctor or j) care for a pregnant family member.

## Office waiting time, recent medical visit

People who had a visit to a physician in the past year were, asked, "How long did you have to wait to see the doctor once you got there?", with respect to their most recent visit.

## Perceived health

"Perceived health" was based on responses to the question, "Would you say your health, in general, is excellent, good, fair or poor?"

## Physician visits

*Saw a physician in the year.* This variable refers to the proportion of the sample who reported at least one physician visit during the survey year.

First, respondents were asked, "What was the month and year of your most recent medical visit when you actually saw a doctor in an office or clinic?" Respondents whose most recent visit was *not* within the last 12 months were then asked, "Did you *see* or *talk* to a doctor any time during the past 12 months, that is since *(Date one year ago)* 1981? This includes visits to the doctor and any visit to a nurse or other medical person on the doctor's staff, instead of the doctor."

*Total visits in the year.* Physician visits include seeing a medical doctor or osteopath or his or her nurse or technician at the following sites: patient's home; doctor's office or private clinic; company or union clinic; school clinic; neighborhood or government-sponsored clinic; hospital outpatient clinic; hospital emergency room; or other place.

Excluded are visits by a doctor to a hospital inpatient. A separate question was asked to elicit whether the respondent talked on the telephone to a doctor or doctor's assistant for prescriptions or medical advice and, if yes, how many times.

*Location of visit.* Visits were reported in terms of the following types of locations: home visit; doctor's office or private clinic; company or union clinic; school clinic; neighborhood or government-sponsored clinic; hospital emergency room; hospital outpatient clinic; or other place.

*Percent hospital emergency room or outpatient clinic visits are of total visits.* This estimate reflects the proportion of visits to a hospital outpatient department or emergency room represent of the total number of visits (excluding phone calls and hospital inpatient contacts) for those who had at least one visit to the doctor in the year.

[See Aday, et al. (1980: 291) for questions used in previous studies.]

## Preventive care

Persons 17 years of age or older were asked if they had a blood pressure reading or had seen a dentist within 12 months of the interview date. Women 17 years of age and older were also asked if they had a Pap smear or a breast exam by a doctor. Proxy respondents for children under 17 years of age were asked if the child ever had a skin test or any kind of test for tuberculosis or TB; an injection or shot against measles; DPT or baby shots; polio shots or medicine; a hearing test, or, within the last 12 months, an eye or dental examination.

## Race

Respondents were asked, "Do you consider yourself White, Black, Oriental or what?" A person was classified as nonwhite if he or she were American Negro, African, West Indian, American Indian, Japanese, Chinese, Filipino, Asian Indian, Korean, Polynesian, Indonesian, Hawaiian, Aleut or Eskimo. Generally, other persons were classified as white. This includes Mexicans, Spaniards and others of Spanish descent.

## Refused care for financial reasons

Adult respondents were asked, "During the last year — since *(Date one year ago)* 1981 — have you or has any member of your family living with you been refused health care because you didn't have insurance or you couldn't pay, or for any other reason?"

## Region

The four regions of the country—Northeast, South, North Central and West—conform to the U.S. Census definitions of those geographic regions.

## Regular source, location

People reporting a regular source of care were asked which of the following places best describes the place they usually go: doctor's office or private clinic, company or union clinic, school or unspecified clinic, neighborhood or government-sponsored clinic, hospital outpatient clinic or unspecified clinic, hospital emergency room, health maintenance organization or other place.

## Regular source, type of

Respondents were asked, "Is there one person or place in particular you usually go to when you are sick or want advice about your health?" Those who said yes were asked, in addition, "Is there one particular doctor you usually see when you go there?" [See Aday, et al. (1980: 294–295) for questions used in 1970 and 1976.]

## Residence

Each telephone number in the 1982 sampling frame contained a code for the geographic area encompassed by the area code exchange. The codes were: 1) central city only; 2) SMSA only; 3) non-SMSA only; 4) central city and SMSA overlap; 5) central city and non-SMSA overlap; 6) central city, SMSA and non-SMSA overlap; and 7) SMSA and non-SMSA overlap. Respondents in categories 4 and 5 were asked, "Do you live in *(Name of city)*, or not?" and respondents in categories 6 and 7 were asked, "What town, city or village do you live in?" Based on the response to either of the two questions, the respondent's residence was then classified in one of the three distinct categories: central city, SMSA outside of central city or non-SMSA.

To ascertain farm status, the interviewer asked, "Do you live on a farm? *(If In Doubt, Ask*: Did you sell $1,000 or more in agricultural products last year?)." Respondents answering "yes" to this question who also live outside of an SMSA were then categorized as living on farms.

[See Aday, et al. (1980: 295–296) for definitions used in previous surveys.]

## Satisfaction with recent visit

These data are available only for persons who had a physician visit during the past year. In addition, the questions were skipped for adult proxy respondents. Seven questions were asked to determine the respondent's satisfaction with different aspects of the visit. For each, the respondent had three choices: "completely satisfied," "somewhat satisfied," and "not at all satisfied."

The aspects about which satisfaction were elicited included a) the amount of time it took to get there; b) the amount of time the person had to wait to see the doctor once there; c) the amount of time the doctor spent with the person; d) the information given to the person about what was wrong with him or her or what was being done to him or her; e) the out-of-pocket cost of the medical care received; f) the quality of the care provided; and g) the overall visit.

[See Aday, et al. (1980: 296) for questions used in 1976.]

## Sex

In those cases in which the interviewer did not specify the sex of a sample person, classification was made on the basis of information provided in the interview.

## Trouble, families in

A family in trouble is one which has had more difficulty getting medical care than in previous years; been refused care; needed but did not get medical help in general or for special services; had a seriously or chronically ill family member and could not find certain services; or had major financial problems due to the illness.

## Would go source, location

People who indicated they did not have a regular source were asked, "Is there a medical doctor or osteopath you *might* go to if you needed medical care?" Those who said "yes" were asked the location of this place. The categories described earlier for the regular source of care were used.

## References

Aday, LuAnn et al. *Health Care in the U.S.: Equitable for Whom?* Beverly Hills, CA: Sage Publications. 1980.

# Appendix D *

## Methodology for Imputing Missing Values, 1982 National Access Survey

Whenever a variety of questions are asked of a large number of survey respondents, it is inevitable that non-responses to specific items will occur in the data. These nonresponses may be due to "refusals" or "don't know" answers or to questions that were inadvertently skipped by the interviewer during the interview. Whatever its source, item nonresponse is a problem in analyzing survey data. Item nonresponse can generally be handled in three ways: 1) calculations can be restricted to only those respondents with complete data; 2) calculations can be restricted to only those variables with valid, reported data, or 3) a missing value imputation procedure can be used

---

*The principal authors of this appendix were Christopher Lyttle, CHAS Programmer/Analyst and Data Manager and Ralph Bell, Ph.D., University Professor, Governors State University.

to estimate what the nonrespondents would have reported had they answered the questions (Frankel and Banks, 1979). The first alternative to handling missing data limits the number of cases on which the analysis is based while the second alternative limits the number and type of variables that can be included in the analysis. Although the third procedure may appear to be the most radical method of handling item nonresponse, we and others have argued that it is in fact the most conservative of the three alternatives (see Bell 1984; Frankel and Banks, 1979; Champney and Bell, 1982a).

The first two methods implicitly assume that the distributions of the missing data are the same as the distributions of the valid data with the same means, medians, etc. (Frankel and Banks, 1979). This assumption may be in error to the extent that individuals who fail to respond to a question are "different" from those who answer the question. The third method allows the distributions of the missing data to vary from those of the valid data and also takes into account the relationships to other data. As a result, the third method is much more likely to produce unbiased estimates of the missing values than the other two alternatives.

In general, imputation methods attempt to provide the best estimates of unreported values in the data by locating a respondent with valid data who has characteristics similar to the respondent who did not answer the question. The valid value from that respondent is then assigned to the missing value for the nonrespondent. In imputation terminology, the respondent with missing data is called the "candidate," and the respondent used to provide the estimated or imputed value is called the "donor." A number of imputation methods have been discussed in the literature. Champney and Bell (1982a; 1982b) have reviewed these alternative imputation procedures and have tested seven different methods to determine which performs best using a quasi-experimental design. The results of this research showed that a modified "hot deck" procedure provides the best estimates of original reported values in continuous data.

However, most of the variables imputed in the present study are categorical. This preferred method was therefore excluded as a possible choice of imputation technique. A modified "bootstrap" procedure (random number generation conditioned by prior distributions on the variable to be imputed) was selected as the next best machine imputation method available. This method is discussed in greater detail later in this appendix. When there were a small number of cases missing on a given variable, and it was deemed important to have only valid values on that variable, case values were imputed by hand. This technique is described below.

## Hand imputation

When a few cases had missing values on variables selected to be imputed, a hand imputation procedure was employed. The process of hand imputation is perhaps the simplest form of imputing data. When a case with a missing value was encountered, we attempted to impute a value for that case which was internally consistent with values reported on other related variables from the same case. An example of this procedure is provided by the following hypothetical situation. Assume that a particular case has a missing value for sex. An examination of the values for several other variables indicates that the head of the household is a male and that the person with the missing data for sex is the spouse of the head of household. Under this simple condition, the respondent is assigned an imputed value for sex indicating female. The imputed value is therefore internally consistent with other variables for that respondent. Although the patterns of nonresponse in the actual data are seldom that straightforward, the principle of imputing for internal consistency is comparable.

## Prior probability random number generation

Imputation by random assignment based on prior distributions is an inexpensive imputation technique particularly appropriate for use when imputing nominal or ordinal variables. This procedure is commonly called a "bootstrap" imputation because in the basic technique only the prior distribution of the variable being imputed is taken into account. We elaborated on this basic technique by defining subgroups relevant to the variable to be imputed that allowed us to make much more accurate estimates of unreported values. The procedure as we used it involves: 1) dividing the cases into cells according to criteria variables relevant to the variable to be imputed; 2) calculating probability ranges for each observed value of the variable to be imputed in the respective cells; 3) generating a random number between zero and one for each case with a missing value, and 4) attaching to the case the observed value in the probability range in which the random number falls. This method, with variation in the definition of cells, was used for imputing 13 variables that were missing on too many cases to make hand imputation a viable alternative. These variables were: Q F7B (farm residence), Q F12 (language of interview), Q F9 (ethnicity), Q F8 (race), Q 10A-Q 10H (visits), and INCPOV (a variable combining income and poverty level).

### Q F7B (farm residence)

Q F7B was imputed in two stages. Cases were imputed in the first stage if they were also missing on Q F2C (occupation of main wage earner). In Stage 1 cases were partitioned into cells based on whether the place they lived was 1) SMSA, central city, 2) SMSA, other or 3) other place. Twenty-two (22) cases were imputed in this stage. In Stage 2 the three categories used in Stage 1 were crossed by whether the main wage earner was a farmer (Q F2C equalled 9) yielding six cells. Fifty (50) cases were imputed in this stage. Overall five residences were imputed to be farms (four in Stage 1 and one in Stage 2). The other cases were assigned a nonfarm status. Distributions before and after imputation show very little change in means or standard deviation for Q F7B (see Table D.1).

## Q F12 (language of interview)

Eight cases were imputed for Q F12. Cells were defined by the values of Q F9 (ethnicity), including a category for missing values on Q F9. All eight interviews were imputed to be in English, and the impact of these few cases on the distribution of the variable was negligible.

## Q F9 (ethnicity)

For Q F9, cells were defined by the values of Q F12 (language of interview) after it had been imputed. This variable is an excellent example of the gain in predictive power for the "bootstrap" method of imputation with the addition of cells defined by criterion variables. Of the cases in the Spanish interview cell, 100 percent were imputed to be of Hispanic origin; of the cases in the English interview cell, 4 percent were imputed to be of Hispanic origin. Overall, 202 cases were imputed. Eleven of these were imputed to be Hispanic. The imputation process produced no significant change in the distribution of the variable.

## Q F8 (race)

Cells were defined for Q F8 by crossing the three categories describing city of residence (see Q F7B, Stage 1 above) with three regions of the country (Northeast and Midwest, South, and West). After imputing 117 cases on race the distribution was shifted slightly in the direction of nonwhites. The reasons for this are better understood by looking at the locations of the imputed cases. The largest concentrations of nonresponse on this item were in SMSA residences in the Northeast, Midwest and West. These are the areas with the largest concentrations of nonwhite population.

## Q 10A thru Q 10H (visits)

Items Q 10A through Q 10H were imputed in two stages. In the first stage cells were defined by the place of usual care (Q 6A). Only those cases indicating on Q 7A that they had a visit within the last year were imputed in this stage. Unfortunately only four cases fell into this category, and so only four cases were imputed in the first stage for each of the visits items. No adequate predictive classifications were available for the remainder of the cases missing on these items. A cell structure was not developed for the second stage of imputation on this variable for that reason. Imputation was based on the original distributions of the respective variables, excluding missing values. The impact of the imputation process on the distributional properties of these items was varied and mostly minor. The largest impact was on item Q 10H (visits to other place), as may be seen in Table D.1.

## INCPOV

This variable is a composite designed specifically to derive both family income and poverty level. In order to develop this variable it was necessary to discard the collapsed income variable provided by Harris, because it deleted some of the poverty cutoff points required in constructing the poverty status variable. Instead we worked with the original income classifications. The cell structure for this variable was defined by crossing the employment status of the main wage earner (Q F2B) by the number of individuals in the family with at least half-time employment (a count of Q D5 within the family). We have reported the prior and post values for the component variables POVLEV and Q F6B (family income) in Table D.1. A total of 507 cases were imputed for these variables.

Table D.1   Means and Standard Deviations
Before and After Imputation*

| Variable | N Imputed | Before Mean | S.D. | After Mean | S.D. |
|---|---|---|---|---|---|
| Q F7B | 72 | 1.9197 | 0.2719 | 1.9198 | 0.2717 |
| Q F12 | 8 | 1.9765 | 0.1516 | 1.9765 | 0.1514 |
| Q F9 | 202 | 1.9239 | 0.2652 | 1.9239 | 0.2651 |
| Q F8 | 117 | 1.1429 | 0.4238 | 1.1451 | 0.4303 |
| Q 10A | 245 | 0.1919 | 2.0393 | 0.1940 | 2.0196 |
| Q 10B | 310 | 4.2071 | 8.3500 | 4.2607 | 8.9582 |
| Q 10C | 251 | 0.1635 | 1.7587 | 0.1610 | 1.7207 |
| Q 10D | 239 | 0.1600 | 1.7246 | 0.1589 | 1.6998 |
| Q 10E | 240 | 0.3411 | 2.2855 | 0.3341 | 2.2405 |
| Q 10F | 254 | 0.7623 | 3.7111 | 0.7625 | 3.6775 |
| Q 10G | 242 | 0.5239 | 1.6960 | 0.5260 | 1.6874 |
| Q 10H | 191 | 4.2976 | 8.1533 | 5.3799 | 10.4819 |
| Q F6B | 507 | 2.4448 | 1.4041 | 2.4352 | 1.4042 |
| POVLEV | 507 | 2.2420 | 0.7999 | 2.2346 | 0.8009 |

*All items here, except the Q 10 variables, are categorical. Means and standard deviations are reported only for descriptive purposes.

## References

Bell, Ralph. "Item Nonresponse in Telephone Surveys: An Analysis of Who Fails to Report Income." *Social Science Quarterly* 65 (March 1984): 205–215.

[a]Champney, Timothy F. and Ralph Bell. "Imputation of Income: A Procedural Comparison." In *Proceedings of the American Statistical Association Section on Survey Research*. Washington, DC: American Statistical Association. 1982.

[b]Champney, Timothy F. and Ralph Bell. "Imputation Procedures: A Comparison Using Hospital Utilization and Expenditure Data." Paper presented at the annual meetings of the American Public Health Association in Montreal, Canada. 1982.

Frankel, Martin R. and Martha J. Banks. "Adjusting for Nonresponse to Specific Questions." In R. Andersen et al. (eds.) *Total Survey Error*. San Francisco, CA: Jossey-Bass. 1979.

# Appendix E *

## Minimum Data Set for Measuring Access to Medical Care

This appendix indicates the questions that should be included on questionnaires designed to measure and monitor access to medical care. In addition, we propose a set of criteria for choosing access measures which have guided our selection of items.

### Criteria for access measures

Measures of access should meet one or more of the following criteria:

A. The measure may be a central measure of one of the key outcome indicators of access defined in the literature (see Aday, et al., 1980: Chapter 1). These include meas-

---

*The principal author of this appendix was Gretchen V. Fleming, Ph.D., Senior Research Associate, CHAS.

ures of utilization, including the more sophisticated need-based measures of utilization, and measures of patient satisfaction. We argue that utilization is the objective proof of access to medical care, whereas patient satisfaction is evidence of subjectively perceived access. "Central measures" are those which reflect the concept as a whole or the most important substantive dimensions of it, such as physician contact rates, volume of physician visits, volume of hospital days and patient satisfaction with overall care or a set of measures of patient satisfaction with the key dimensions of care.

B. A measure of access may be chosen because it has been traditionally used; therefore data are already available for tracing patterns over time. A somewhat imprecise measure which has been used in a number of previous studies may be valuable if we believe that the percent of "error" in the measure has remained constant over time. It is always difficult to choose between refining a measure and keeping a cruder measure that is more comparable to earlier data. In this "minimum" data set we have had to make this choice in several instances.

C. Some measures are chosen because they have proven in earlier work to be highly sensitive measures of "potential" access, or *predictors* of key access outcomes (see Aday, et al., 1980: Chapter 2). For instance, such measures as having or not having a regular source of care and insurance coverage may be viewed as potential access indicators but, within our framework, in themselves, they are not proof that access was realized. Rather they either facilitate or impede actual (realized) access. These measures for the most part describe the respondent's relationship to the medical care system in terms of experiences other than actual utilization rates and satisfaction with care.

D. Finally, some measures may be chosen because we may expect to see a change in them due to current policy initiatives. For instance, changes in reimbursement of hospital stays based on diagnosis rather than length of stay may lead to shorter lengths of stay for patients in the hospital, with more admissions on average per year. Therefore, average number of hospital admissions may become an even more important measure to monitor over time.

## Independent variables

The above measures address the criteria for choosing both "potential" and "realized" indicators of access. The minimum data set for measuring access should also include key independent or predictor variables, although additional measures may be desired depending on the population being sampled and the goals of a given study. Of the proposed set, most of these variables would be required in any study of the health care of the U.S. population. The measures of need are considered crucial for measuring access in any population. The criteria for selecting the independent variables parallel those for the access outcomes. They are as follows:

A. For the access outcomes we argued above that certain central measures of the concept should always be included. The argument for certain independent variables is similar. Measures of need are central in this case. They are absolutely essential for standardizing the data base so that we may compare levels of appropriate access across population groups and over time. These measures include patient perceptions of illness as well as physician-diagnosed illness. Measures of age and sex should also be included as proxies for kinds of "need" which may not be adequately described in other measures.

B. In addition, as with the access outcome measures, certain traditional independent variables should be included because they permit us to monitor access for policy relevant subgroups over time. These include place of residence, racial/ethnic breakdowns, income and education.

C. We should also include independent variables which have been shown to be sensitive predictors of key access measures. The need measures as well as race and poverty levels fit this criterion as do other measures.

D. Finally, as with the potential and realized access measures, we wish to include independent variables that describe population groups for which we expect to see access changes due to recent policy initiatives. For instance, as programs for the poor (such as Medicaid) change in form, we might expect to see the access of the poor altered. In addition, we wish to identify subgroups whose experience may drive overall trends. For instance, fluctuations in the unemployment rate could lead to corresponding increases or decreases in doctor contact rates and volume of visits.

## Application of criteria

It is clear that many access measures and independent variables may meet more than one criterion for inclusion. In addition there is at least one important further distinction to be made in these criteria. Criteria A, B and C define measures we would expect to see in the minimum data set gathered to measure access over the long term. Criterion D, on the other hand, describes a changing subset of measures, attuned to current policy initiatives and hypotheses about how they may affect the population. In other words, the minimum data set has a dynamic quality in that it must change to reflect societal changes and changes in the medical care system in particular.

The minimum data set is described in Tables E.1 and E.2, Access Questions and Independent Variables, respectively. The choice of questions is predicated on the assumption of a telephone or household survey. Where the form of the question would change depending on which of these two survey modes is used, some indication is given of a source for identifying appropriate question alterations. The minimum data set is also relevant to a questionnaire that the respondent would fill out, but needed adjustments required in the questionnaire format are not described here. In addition, because of many possible variations in sample design, we have not made an effort to include questions that might be needed to properly handle sampling issues, such as for the proper weighting of cases. These would need to be added.

Wording of most access measures is provided in Table E.1. However, readers are advised to look at the original questionnaires and consult experts at interview formatting prior to constructing a questionnaire with these items, as this will help in laying out response categories and suggesting interviewer probes. In Table E.2, where we have listed the independent variables, we have referenced the versions of questions that should be used from the 1982 and/or 1976 survey instruments. The 1982 instrument is reproduced in Appendix F, and the 1976 instrument may be found in Aday, et al., 1980: Appendix G. Where 1976 versions of questions are suggested, it is because there were methodological problems with the versions in the 1982 instruments.

## References

Aday, LuAnn et al. *Health Care in the U.S. Equitable for Whom?* Beverly Hills, CA: Sage Publications. 1980.

## TABLE E.1 Access Questions

| QUESTION NUMBER FROM 1982 ACCESS SURVEY | QUESTIONS AND COMMENTS | CRITERION MET |
|---|---|---|
| 3a | How many days altogether during the past year, that is, since (DATE ONE YEAR AGO), did you (s/he) stay in bed more than half of the day because of illness or injury? Include any days you (s/he) stayed in the hospital.<br><br>COMMENT: THIS QUESTION AND Q. 3b ARE COMPONENTS OF THE USE-DISABILITY RATIO. | A,B |
| 3b | Not counting the days in bed, how many days during the past year, that is, since (DATE ONE YEAR AGO), did you (s/he), have to cut down on the things you usually do (s/he usually does) for more than half of the day because of illness or injury?<br><br>COMMENT: SEE COMMENT FOR 3a. | A,B |
| 4a | PREFERRED WORDING IS FROM 1976 ACCESS STUDY AS POSITIVE ANSWERS MAY HAVE BEEN SLIGHTLY OVERSTATED HERE:<br><br>"Have you had any of the following tests this past year, that is since (DATE ONE YEAR AGO)?<br><br>a. Blood pressure reading" | D |
| 4b | PREFERRED WORDING IS FROM 1976 ACCESS STUDY AS POSITIVE ANSWERS MAY HAVE BEEN OVERSTATED:<br><br>"About how long has it been since you were last treated or examined by a dentist?" | A,B |
| 4c | PREFERRED WORDING IS FROM 1976 ACCESS STUDY (SEE 4a ABOVE FOR COMMENT AND BASIC QUESTION):<br><br>"b. A Pap smear test for cancer?" | D |
| 4d | SEE NOTE FOR 4c:<br><br>"c. A breast examination by a doctor?" | D |

# TABLE E.1 (continued)  Access Questions

| | | |
|---|---|---|
| 5a | Is there one person or place in particular you (s/he) usually go(es) to when you are (s/he is) sick or (s/he) want(s) advice about your (her/his) health? | B,C |
| 5c | Is there a medical doctor or osteopath you (s/he) <u>might</u> go to if you (s/he) needed medical care? | C |
| 6a | Where do you (does s/he) usually go—to a doctor's office, a clinic, a hospital, or some other place? | B,C |
| | PROBE WITH A, B, OR C BEFORE RECORDING. | |
| | A.  IF CLINIC:  Is it a private clinic; a hospital outpatient clinic; a company or union clinic; a school clinic; a neighborhood or government-sponsored clinic; or any other clinic not connected with a hospital? | |
| | B.  IF HOSPITAL:  Is it a hospital outpatient clinic or a hospital emergency room? | |
| | C.  IF SOME OTHER PLACE:  What type of place is it? | |
| 6c | Is there one particular doctor you (s/he) usually see(s) when you (s/he) go(es) there? | B,C |
| 7a | What was the month and year of your (her/his) most recent medical visit—when you (s/he) actually saw a doctor in an office or at a clinic? | A |
| | COMMENT:  THIS QUESTION SHOULD FOLLOW Q.8 RATHER THAN SERVE AS SCREENER QUESTION, ITSELF, FOR USE IN PAST YEAR. HOWEVER, IT IS USEFUL FOR GETTING PEOPLE TO FOCUS ON THEIR LAST VISIT. ABOUT WHICH WE ARE GOING TO ASK THE NEXT FEW QUESTIONS. | |
| 7b | To what type of place did you (s/he) go for this last visit--did you (s/he) go to a doctor's office, a clinic, a hospital, or some other place? | A |
| | COMMENT:  SEE COMMENT FOR 7a. | |
| 7f | How long did you (s/he) have to wait to see the doctor once you (s/he) got there? | C |

## TABLE E.1 (continued)  Access Questions

7g  During your last visit for medical care, were you completely satisfied        A
    somewhat satisfied, or not at all satisfied with (READ EACH ITEM)?

    a.  The amount of time it took you to get there.....

    b.  The amount of time you had to wait to see the doctor, once there...

    c.  The amount of time the doctor spent with you.......

    d.  The information given to you about what was wrong with you, or about
        what was being done for you.....

    e.  The out-of-pocket cost for the medical care received, that is, the
        cost not paid by insurance..........

    f.  The quality of care you felt was provided at that visit.......

    ASK ITEM "g" LAST

    g.  The visit to the doctor, overall..........

    COMMENT:  IT WOULD BE PREFERABLE TO USE A SCALE WITH 5 POINTS.
              HOWEVER SUCH A SCALE THAT WILL WORK BY TELEPHONE HAS NOT BEEN USED
              IN A NATIONAL STUDY OF ACCESS, SO IT IS PROBABLY BETTER TO
              USE THE HARRIS 1982 STUDY SCALE TO BEGIN TO MEASURE TRENDS.
              RECOGNIZING THAT MEASURES SHOULD THEN BE DICHOTOMIZED AND
              TREATED SEPARATELY.

8   Did you (s/he) see or talk to a doctor any time during the past              A,B
    twelve months, that is since (DATE ONE YEAR AGO)? This includes
    visits to the doctor and any visit to a nurse or other medical person
    on the doctor's staff, instead of the doctor.

    COMMENT:  EXACT WORDING SHOULD BE FOLLOWED: MEASURE VERY SENSITIVE TO
              INCLUSION OF NURSE VISITS.

## TABLE E.1 (continued) Access Questions

| | | |
|---|---|---|
| 10 | How many of each of the following kinds of visits did you (s/he) have with a doctor or doctor's assistant during the past twelve months, that is, since (DATE ONE YEAR AGO)? | A,B |
| | House calls by a doctor or doctor's assistant..... | |
| | Visits to a doctor's office or private clinic........ | |
| | Visits to a company or union clinic.......... | |
| | Visits to a school clinic........ | |
| | Visits to a neighborhood or government-sponsored clinic.... | |
| | Visits to a hospital outpatient clinic.......... | |
| | Visits to a hospital emergency room........ | |
| | Visits to any other place for medical care, other than when you may have been a patient overnight in a hospital (SPECIFY) | |
| 11a | Did you (s/he) talk on the telephone to a doctor or doctor's assistant for prescriptions or medical advice any time during the past twelve months, that is, since (DATE ONE YEAR AGO)? | D |
| 11b | How many times did you (s/he) talk on the telephone to a doctor or doctor's assistant for prescriptions or medical advice? | D |
| 17a | Have you (has s/he) been a patient overnight in a hospital during the past twelve months, since (DATE ONE YEAR AGO)? | A,B |
| 17b | How many times were you (was s/he) admitted to a hospital since (DATE ONE YEAR AGO)? | D |
| 17c | Altogether, how many nights did you (s/he) stay in a hospital during that period, that is since (DATE ONE YEAR AGO)? | A,B |

# TABLE E.1 (continued) Access Questions

22  Now I'd like to talk about the different kinds of health plans or health insurance that people have, including those provided by the government. As I read each of the following health plans, please tell me whether you are (s/he is) covered by it. READ EACH ITEM

B.C

Health insurance through work or union......

Health insurance through some other group......

Health insurance bought directly by yourself (herself/himself) or your (her/his) family......

Medicare A, that pays hospital bills for people aged 65 and over and for some disabled people......

Medicare B, that pays doctor's bills for people aged 65 and over and and for some disabled people......

Medicaid or Public Aid......

Prepaid group practice or an HMO (that is, a place you go for all or most medical care which is paid for by a fixed monthly or annual amount)(USE PROBE BELOW)......

Another clinic or health care center where you (s/he) can get care at no cost or at reduced rates......

Any other place? (SPECIFY) (IF RESPONDENT SAYS "BLUE CROSS" OR "BLUE SHIELD" OR NAMES A SPECIFIC INSURANCE COMPANY, USE PROBE BELOW AND DO NOT RECORD HERE.)

PROBE:  Was it purchased through work or a union, through some other group, brought directly by yourself (herself/himself), or the family, or purchased some other way?

COMMENT:  THIS SHOULD BE ASKED FOR EVERYONE, INCLUDING CHILDREN, WHICH WAS NOT DONE IN THE 1982 ACCESS SURVEY.

23  Does your (her/his) health insurance coverage pay part, all, or none of the cost of (READ EACH ITEM)?

A.B

a.  Visits to the doctor's office......

b.  Hospital expenses......

c.  Surgical expenses......

d.  Prescribed medicine taken outside of the hospital......

A.B

SYMPTOMS-RESPONSE RATIO QUESTION AND NORMS, NOT USED IN 1982 ACCESS SURVEY, IS A KEY MEASURE. SEE ADAY, ET AL., 1980: APPENDIX E AND APPENDIX G, Q.35, FOR COMPONENTS. CHAS HAS ALSO DEVELOPED A TELEPHONE VERSION OF THIS QUESTION FOR THE MUNICIPAL HEALTH SERVICES PROGRAM EVALUATION.

# TABLE E.2 Independent Variables

| QUESTION REFERENCE (a) | VARIABLES | | CRITERION MET |
|---|---|---|---|
| 1976: HOUSEHOLD ENUMERATION FOLDER Q 1-14 | AGE, SEX, MARITAL STATUS, FAMILY SIZE | | B,C,D |
| | COMMENT: | PORTION OF Q.1 IN THIS MODEL THAT SAYS, "who are related to the head of the household", SHOULD BE OMITTED IN THE MINIMUM DATA SET. INSTEAD, PERSONS MAY BE LISTED IN AGE ORDER, AFTER THE RESPONDENT. IF SAMPLING IS TO BE DONE FROM THIS LIST. THUS QUESTION WORDING SHOULD BE CHANGED SLIGHTLY TO REFLECT THESE CHANGES. | |
| 1982: F1b, F2a, F2b | MAIN WAGE EARNER EDUCATION, EMPLOYMENT STATUS | | B,C,D |
| | COMMENT: | EDUCATION MAY BE RECORDED SIMPLY AS A CONTINUOUS VARIABLE. | |
| 1976: 154, 155 | INCOME | | B,C,D |
| | COMMENT: | CHAS HAS ALSO DEVELOPED A TELEPHONE VERSION OF THIS QUESTION FOR THE MUNICIPAL HEALTH SERVICES PROGRAM EVALUATION. A CATEGORIZED VERSION OF THE INCOME QUESTION SHOULD FOLLOW THE CONTINUOUS VERSION OF THE QUESTION SUGGESTED HERE FOR THOSE WHO REFUSE THE CONTINUOUS VERSION. HOWEVER, THE CONTINUOUS ITEM SHOULD BE ASKED FIRST SO AS TO HAVE FINER DATA ON INCOME TO BE USED IN CREATING POVERTY-LEVEL CUTOFFS FOR DIFFERENT FAMILY SIZES AND RESIDENTIAL SETTINGS. FROM THE RELATIVELY FEW CATEGORIZED RESPONSES "CONTINUOUS" DATA CAN BE ESTIMATED OR IMPUTED. | |
| 1982: F7b, F7c, F7d | RESIDENCE | | B,C,D |
| | COMMENT: | THESE QUESTIONS WILL VARY DEPENDING ON SAMPLING CHARACTERISTICS. HOWEVER, Q F7b IS APPROPRIATE WHEREVER FARM FAMILIES NEED TO BE IDENTIFIED FOR CONSISTENCY WITH THIS AND EARLIER DATA. | |
| 1982: F8, F9 | RACE/ETHNICITY | | B,C,D |
| 1982: 2 | PERCEIVED HEALTH | | A,B,C |
| 1982: 35, 36, 37a, 37b | CHRONIC ILLNESS | | A,C,D |
| 1982: 3a, 3b | DISABILITY DAYS: SEE COMMENTS ON WORDING FOR ITEM IN TABLE E.1. HOWEVER THESE ARE ALSO KEY MEASURES OF NEED. | | A,B,C |

(a) 1982: (Question number) refers to a question on the 1982 Access Survey (See Appendix F).
    1976: (Question number) refers to a question on the 1976 Access Survey (Aday, et al., 1980: Appendix G).

# Appendix F
## The Questionnaire

LOUIS HARRIS AND ASSOCIATES, INC.
630 Fifth Avenue
New York, New York  10111

Study No. 824002

April 1982          (9-10)      Sample Point No._____
                                 11-12-13-14-15-16-17-18-19-20-21-22

Cross Section               **01**
                           (23 - 24)

Interviewer:_____Date:_____

Telephone No._____

--------------------------------------------------------------------------

Hello, I'm _____from Louis Harris and Associates, the public
opinion research company.  We're talking to people all over the country about health
care issues facing the public.  We're interested in learning more about the medical care
that  people need for themselves and their families.  I'd like to talk about your
experiences in getting medical care when you need it.  First, I need to ask a few
general questions to see if we can include you in our survey.  Are you 17 years of age
or older?  (IF NO, ASK TO SPEAK WITH SOMEONE 17 YEARS OF AGE OR OLDER.)

--------------------------------------------------------------------------

S1a.  Including yourself, how many adults 17 years of age and older in your family live
in this home or living quarters?  Please include people who are temporarily in the
hospital or who may have entered a nursing home or any other health or convalescent
facility in the last six months.

INTERVIEWER NOTE:  IF PERSON ON PHONE DOES NOT LIVE THERE, ASK:  May I speak to
                   someone who lives here?

S1b.  How many of the adults are females?
RECORD Q.S1a AND Q.S1b ON GRID A

### VERSION I

#### Circle Number of Adults In Family

| | | 1 | 2 | 3 | 4 | 5 | 6 + |
|---|---|---|---|---|---|---|---|
| | O | MALE | YOUNGER MALE | 2ND YOUNGEST MALE | 2ND YOUNGEST MALE | 2ND YOUNGEST MALE | 4TH OLDEST MALE |
| Circle Number | 1 | FEMALE | MALE | OLDEST MALE | 2ND YOUNGEST MALE | 2ND YOUNGEST MALE | 3rd OLDEST MALE |
| of Adult | 2 | | YOUNGER FEMALE | YOUNGEST FEMALE | OLDEST MALE | 2ND YOUNGEST MALE | 2ND OLDEST MALE |
| Females | 3 | | | 2ND YOUNGEST FEMALE | YOUNGEST FEMALE | OLDER MALE | OLDEST MALE |
| | 4 | | | | 2ND YOUNGEST FEMALE | YOUNGEST FEMALE | YOUNGEST FEMALE |
| | 5 | | | | | 2ND YOUNGEST FEMALE | 2ND YOUNGEST FEMALE |
| | 6 + | | | | | | 4TH OLDEST FEMALE |

(25)

S1c.  Could you give me the first name or initials of (DESIGNATED RESPONDENT IN GRID A)?
RECORD NAME FOR "ADULT DESIGNATED RESPONDENT" AT BOTTOM OF PAGE 1

INTERVIEWER:.  "X" FINAL INTERVIEW STATUS.
              ADULT/ADULT PROXY COMPLETED...(27(_____-1
              ADULT/ADULT PROXY NOT COMPLETED..._____-2
              NO CHILD PROXY REQUIRED.........._____-3
              CHILD PROXY COMPLETED............._____-4
              CHILD PROXY NOT COMPLETED........._____-5

(262)

-1-    CARD 01    824002

S2a.  And how many children under the age of 17 in your family live in your home or living quarters?  Please include any infants and children temporarily in the hospital or any other health or convalescent facility.

IF NONE, RECORD BELOW AND SKIP TO Q.S3.
IF ANY CHILDREN, RECORD ON GRID B AND ASK Q.S2b.

No children in family.........(28(    -1

S2b.  How many of them are girls?
RECORD ON GRID B

| VERSION I | | | | | |
|---|---|---|---|---|---|
| Circle Number of Children In Family | | | | | |
| 1 | 2 | 3 | 4 | 5 | 6 + |

|  | | 1 | 2 | 3 | 4 | 5 | 6 + |
|---|---|---|---|---|---|---|---|
| Circle Number | O | MALE | YOUNGER MALE | 2ND YOUNGEST MALE | 2ND YOUNGEST MALE | 2ND YOUNGEST MALE | 4TH OLDEST MALE |
| of | 1 | FEMALE | MALE | OLDEST MALE | 2ND YOUNGEST MALE | 2ND YOUNGEST MALE | 3RD OLDEST MALE |
| Female | 2 | | YOUNGER FEMALE | YOUNGEST FEMALE | OLDEST MALE | 2ND YOUNGEST MALE | 2ND OLDEST MALE |
|  | 3 | | | 2ND YOUNGEST FEMALE | YOUNGEST FEMALE | OLDER MALE | OLDEST MALE |
| Children | 4 | | | | 2ND YOUNGEST FEMALE | YOUNGEST FEMALE | YOUNGEST FEMALE |
|  | 5 | | | | | 2ND YOUNGEST FEMALE | 2ND YOUNGEST FEMALE |
|  | 6 + | | | | | | 4TH OLDEST FEMALE |

(29)

S2c.  Which adult in the family knows the most about the health care for (CHILD SELECTED BY GRID B)?
RECORD NAME BELOW FOR "CHILD PROXY"

S3.  (IF "ADULT DESIGNATED RESPONDENT" OR "CHILD PROXY" IS ALREADY ON THE PHONE, CONDUCT THAT INTERVIEW FIRST.  IF NEITHER ON PHONE, ASK: I need to interview (ADULT DESIGNATED RESPONDENT) and (CHILD PROXY)).  Is either of them home now?

IF ONE RESPONDENT HOME, CONDUCT APPROPRIATE INTERVIEW AND MAKE APPOINTMENT OR FIND OUT THE BEST TIME TO CALL BACK FOR THE OTHER INTERVIEW.

IF NEITHER IS HOME, GET NAMES FOR BOTH RESPONDENTS AND MAKE APPOINTMENTS OR FIND OUT BEST TIME TO CALL BACK.

IF ADULT DESIGNATED RESPONDENT IS IN THE HOSPITAL, A NURSING HOME, OR IS INCAPACITATED BY ILLNESS, OR ADULT SELECTED BY GRID DOES NOT SPEAK ENGLISH OR SPANISH, ASK TO SPEAK TO ADULT WHO IS THE MOST KNOWLEDGEABLE ABOUT THAT PERSON'S HEALTH CARE.  RECORD NAME BELOW FOR "PROXY FOR ADULT."

RECORD RESPONDENT NAME(S)                    BEST TIME TO CALL BACK:

_____    _____
Adult Designated Respondent

_____    _____
Child Proxy

_____    _____
Proxy for adult in hospital, nursing home, or incapacitated by illness.

ASK OF FIRST QUALIFIED RESPONDENT:
D1. (INTERVIEWER:  RECORD NAMES OF ADULT DESIGNATED RESPONDENT OR ADULT PROXY, AND
CHILD PROXY, IF DIFFERENT PERSON, AS "1" AND "2" ON GRID BELOW.)  First, I need to get a
few details about each member of your family.  I've already gotten (NAMES OF ADULT
DR/PROXY, CHILD PROXY) written down.  Now, starting with the oldest, please give me the
first name of each of the other members of the family who live in this household,
including any who are now away at school and who live in a dormitory there.  (RECORD ON
GRID BELOW BEGINNING WITH "3.")

IF NAME REFUSED, PROBE FOR POSITION IN HOUSEHOLD.

ASK Q.D2-D5 CONSECUTIVELY FOR EACH FAMILY MEMBER
D2. (RECORD SEX FOR EACH HOUSEHOLD MEMBER LISTED IN Q.D1.  IF NECESSARY, PROBE.)

D3. How old are you (is s/he)?  (IF REFUSED OR NOT SURE, PROBE:  Are you (is s/he)
between the ages of 17-20, 21-24, 25-29, 30-34, 35-39, 40-49, 50-64, or are you (is
s/he) 65 or over?)
RECORD 2-DIGIT NUMBER FOR EACH BELOW.  IF REFUSED, RECORD 97, IF NOT SURE, RECORD 98.
IF LESS THAN 1 YEAR, RECORD 00

ASK Q.D4-D5 ONLY FOR ADULT FAMILY MEMBERS 17 YEARS OF AGE AND OLDER

D4. Are you (is s/he) married, widowed, divorced, separated, or single?
RECORD BELOW FOR EACH ADULT

D5. Do you (does s/he) work at least 15 hours a week, or not?
RECORD BELOW FOR EACH ADULT

| Q.D1 Name/Position | Q.D2 Sex Male | Female | Q.D3 Age (Write In) | Q.D4 Marital Status Married | Wid- owed | Div- orced | Separ- ated | Single | Refused | Q.D5 Work Yes | No | Refused |
|---|---|---|---|---|---|---|---|---|---|---|---|---|
| 01 (Adult DR) | (11( __-1 | __-2 | (12-13) | (14( __-1 | __-2 | __-3 | __-4 | __-5 | __-7 | (15( __-1 | __-2 | __-7 |
| 02 (Child Proxy) | (16( __-1 | __-2 | (17-18) | (19( __-1 | __-2 | __-3 | __-4 | __-5 | __-7 | (20( __-1 | __-2 | __-7 |
| 03 | (21( __-1 | __-2 | (22-23) | (24( __-1 | __-2 | __-3 | __-4 | __-5 | __-7 | (25( __-1 | __-2 | __-7 |
| 04 | (26( __-1 | __-2 | (27-28) | (29( __-1 | __-2 | __-3 | __-4 | __-5 | __-7 | (30( __-1 | __-2 | __-7 |
| 05 | (31( __-1 | __-2 | (32-33) | (34( __-1 | __-2 | __-3 | __-4 | __-5 | __-7 | (35( __-1 | __-2 | __-7 |
| 06 | (36( __-1 | __-2 | (37-38) | (39( __-1 | __-2 | __-3 | __-4 | __-5 | __-7 | (40( __-1 | __-2 | __-7 |
| 07 | (41( __-1 | __-2 | (42-43) | (44( __-1 | __-2 | __-3 | __-4 | __-5 | __-7 | (45( __-1 | __-2 | __-7 |
| 08 | (46( __-1 | __-2 | (47-48) | (49( __-1 | __-2 | __-3 | __-4 | __-5 | __-7 | (50( __-1 | __-2 | __-7 |
| 09 | (51( __-1 | __-2 | (52-53) | (54( __-1 | __-2 | __-3 | __-4 | __-5 | __-7 | (55( __-1 | __-2 | __-7 |
| 10 | (56( __-1 | __-2 | (57-58) | (59( __-1 | __-2 | __-3 | __-4 | __-5 | __-7 | (60( __-1 | __-2 | __-7 |
| 11 | (61( __-1 | __-2 | (62-63) | (64( __-1 | __-2 | __-3 | __-4 | __-5 | __-7 | (65( __-1 | __-2 | __-7 |
| 12 | (66( __-1 | __-2 | (67-68) | (69( __-1 | __-2 | __-3 | __-4 | __-5 | __-7 | (70( __-1 | __-2 | __-7 |

(01-02)

INTERVIEWER:  CHECK NUMBER OF ADULTS AND CHILDREN, AND NUMBER OF FEMALES IN EACH
CATEGORY, AGAINST RESPONSES IN Q.S1a, S1b, S2a, S2b.

D6. INTERVIEWER:  RECORD 2-DIGIT CODE FROM Q.D1 FOR CHILD DESIGNATED IN GRID B.  PROBE
IF NECESSARY.

(71-72)

-3-    CARD 01    824002

D7. Are any of the people you have named away at school and living in a dormitory? (IF YES, ASK:) Who? |RECORD 2-DIGIT CODES FROM Q.D1.|

(73-74)  (75-76)  (77-78)  (79-80)

| IF SPEAKING TO DESIGNATED RESPONDENT GO TO Q.1a IN MAIN QUESTIONNAIRE.
| IF SPEAKING TO CHILD PROXY, GO TO Q.42 IN MAIN QUESTIONNAIRE.

| ALL FACTUALS ARE TO BE ASKED AT THE END OF THE FIRST INTERVIEW CONDUCTED AT EACH
| HOUSEHOLD

F1a. INTERVIEWER: RECORD, DO NOT ASK:
     PERSON ANSWERING FACTUALS IS:

                    Adult designated respondent.....(30(____-1
                    Adult proxy.........................____-2
                    Child proxy.........................____-3
                    Refused.............................____-7
                    Not sure/don't know.................____-8
                    No answer/interviewer error.........____-9

F1b. Who is the main wage earner or provider of income in your family?

| INTERVIEWER: IF RESPONDENT SAYS MORE THAN ONE WAGE EARNER, PROBE FOR HOUSEHOLD
| MEMBER WITH HIGHEST INCOME.

                    _____    (31-32)
                    RECORD NAME OR POSITION

| INTERVIEWER: CHECK GRID ON PAGE 2 AND RECORD: |

                    Main wage earner is adult designated
                       respondent in Grid on Page 2.........(33(____-1  (SKIP TO Q.F3a)

                    Main wage earner is not adult
                       designated respondent in Grid on Page 2...____-2  (ASK Q.F2a)

| ASK Q.F2a, F2b, F2c FOR ADULT DESIGNATED RESPONDENT IN GRID ON PAGE 2 IF NOT
| A MAIN WAGE EARNER.

F2a. What was the last grade of school that the main wage earner (PERSON IN Q.F1b) completed?

                    No formal schooling.........(34(____-1
                    First through 7th grade.........____-2
                    8th grade.......................____-3
                    Some high school................____-4
                    High school graduate............____-5
                    Some college....................____-6
                    Two-year college graduate.......____-7
                    Four-year college graduate......____-8
                    Postgraduate....................____-9
                    Trade/technical/vocational
                       after high school*..........XXXXXX
                    Refused.....................(35(____-7
                    Not sure/don't know.............____-8
                    No answer/interviewer error.....____-9

| *INTERVIEWER: ASK FOR DETAILS, AND CODE INTO ONE OF THE ABOVE CATEGORIES. |

F2b.  Which of the following best describes (her/his) current employment situation:  Is (s/he) (READ LIST)?

```
         a.  Working full-time.................(36(    -1 ⎞
         b.  Working part-time.....................    -2 ⎪
         c.  Laid off or on strike.................    -3 ⎬ (ASK Q.F2c)
         d.  Unemployed but looking for work.......    -4 ⎪
         e.  Unemployed and not looking for work...    -5 ⎠

         f.  Retired.............................    -6 ⎞
         g.  Unable to work -- disabled...........    -7 ⎬ (SKIP TO Q.F3a)
         h.  Keeping house........................    -8 ⎪
         i.  Full-time student....................    -9 ⎠

             Refused..........................(37(    -7 ⎞
             Not sure/don't know...................    -8 ⎬ (ASK Q.F2c)
             No answer/interviewer error..........    -9 ⎠
```

F2c.  What type of work does (s/he) (PERSON IN Q.F1b) do?

```
+-----------------------------------------------------------------------+
|                        DESCRIBE JOB BRIEFLY:                          |
|                                                                       |
|                                                                       |
+-----------------------------------------------------------------------+
```

```
         Professional..............................(38(    -1
         Manager, official.............................     -2
         Proprietor (small business)....................    -3
         Clerical worker................................    -4
         Sales worker...................................    -5
         Skilled craftsman, foreman.....................    -6
         Operative, unskilled laborer (except farm).....    -7
         Service worker.................................    -8
         Farmer, farm manager, farm laborer.............    -9
         Military service.........................(39(    -1
         Other (SPECIFY)

         _____ ..____    -2
         Refused........................................    -7
         Not sure/don't know............................    -8
         No answer/interviewer error....................    -9
```

F3a.  What was the last grade of school that you (s/he) completed?

```
         No formal schooling........(40(    -1
         First through 7th grade.........    -2
         8th grade.......................    -3
         Some high school................    -4
         High school graduate............    -5
         Some college....................    -6
         Two-year college graduate.......    -7
         Four-year college graduate......    -8
         Postgraduate....................    -9
         Trade/technical/vocational
           after high school*...........XXXXXX
         Refused....................(41(    -7
         Not sure/don't know.............    -8
         No answer/interviewer error.....    -9
```

*INTERVIEWER:  ASK FOR DETAILS, AND CODE INTO ONE OF THE ABOVE CATEGORIES.

-5-          CARD 01                    824002

F3b.  Which of the following best describes your (her/his) current employment
situation?  |READ LIST|

                    a.  Working full-time.................(42(____-1 ⎫
                    b.  Working part-time.....................____-2 ⎬
                    c.  Laid off or on strike................____-3 ⎬(ASK Q.F3c)
                    d.  Unemployed but looking for work.......____-4 ⎬
                    e.  Unemployed and not looking for work...____-5 ⎭

                    f.  Retired.............................____-6 ⎫
                    g.  Unable to work -- disabled...........____-7 ⎬(SKIP TO Q.F4a)
                    h.  Keeping house........................____-8 ⎬
                    i.  Full-time student....................____-9 ⎭

                    Refused...........................(43(____-7 ⎫
                    Not sure/don't know. ..................____-8 ⎬(ASK Q.F3c)
                    No answer/interviewer error...........____-9 ⎭

F3c.  What type of work do you (does s/he) do?

| DESCRIBE JOB BRIEFLY: |
| --- |
|  |

                    Professional............................(44(____-1
                    Manager, official..........................____-2
                    Proprietor (small business)................____-3
                    Clerical worker............................____-4
                    Sales worker...............................____-5
                    Skilled craftsman, foreman.................____-6
                    Operative, unskilled laborer (except farm).____-7
                    Service worker.............................____-8
                    Farmer, farm manager, farm laborer.........____-9
                    Military service.......................(45(____-1
                    Other (SPECIFY) _____
                    _____ .._____-2
                    Refused....................................____-7
                    Not sure/don't know........................____-8
                    No answer/interviewer error................____-9

|ASK EVERYONE|
F4a.  Does anyone in your family receive AFDC, Aid for Families with Dependent Children,
or not?

                    Yes, someone receives.......(46(____-1
                    No, no one receives.............____-2
                    Refused.........................____-7
                    Not sure/don't know.............____-8
                    No answer/interviewer error......____-9

F4b.  Does anyone in your family receive SSI, Supplemental Security Income, or not?

                    Yes, someone receives.......(47(____-1
                    No, no one receives.............____-2
                    Refused.........................____-7
                    Not sure/don't know.............____-8
                    No answer/interviewer error......____-9

F5a.  In the last year have the earnings of your family been reduced by a health problem
or disability of a wage earner or not?

                    Yes, have been reduced......(48(____-1  (ASK Q.F5b)

                    No, have not....................____-2 ⎫
                    Not sure/refused................____-3 ⎬
                    Refused.........................____-7 ⎬(SKIP TO Q.F6a)
                    Not sure/don't know.............____-8 ⎬
                    No answer/interviewer error.....____-9 ⎭

-6-        CARD  01          824002

F5b.  Has the income of your family been seriously reduced, reduced somewhat, or reduced a little because of the illness of a wage earner?

Seriously reduced.........(49(    -1
Reduced somewhat...............____ -2
Reduced a little...............____ -3
Refused........................____ -7
Not sure/don't know...........____ -8
No answer/interviewer error....____ -9

F6a.  Can I just confirm, how many people in your family, including yourself -- adults and children -- live in your home or living quarters?
|CIRCLE RESPONSE ON TOP LINE OF GRID BELOW|

F6b.  Which of the following income categories best describes your total 1981 family income?  Please be sure to include income from welfare, Social Security, pensions, and investments, as well as any wages and salary or income from your own business.
|READ INCOME CATEGORIES IN COLUMN UNDERNEATH NUMBER CIRCLED ON GRID BELOW, AND RECORD.|

NUMBER IN FAMILY IN Q.F6a:  (CIRCLE)

| 1 | 2 | 3 |
|---|---|---|
| $4,700 or less...(50(   -1 | $6,100 or less...(52(   -1 | $7,200 or less...(54(   -1 |
| $4,701-7,200.........____ -2 | $6,101-7,200.........____ -2 | $7,201-10,900.......____ -2 |
| $7,201-15,000.......____ -3 | $7,201-9,200.........____ -3 | $10,901-15,000......____ -3 |
| $15,001-25,000......____ -4 | $9,201-15,000.......____ -4 | $15,001-25,000......____ -4 |
| $25,001-35,000......____ -5 | $15,001-25,000......____ -5 | $25,001-35,000......____ -5 |
| $35,001-50,000......____ -6 | $25,001-35,000......____ -6 | $35,001-50,000......____ -6 |
| Over $50,000.........____ -7 | $35,001-50,000......____ -7 | Over $50,000.........____ -7 |
| Refused..........(51(   -7 | Over $50,000.........____ -8 | Refused..........(55(   -7 |
| Not sure/don't know..____ -8 | Refused..........(53(   -7 | Not sure/don't know..____ -8 |
| No answer/ | Not sure/don't know..____ -8 | No answer/ |
|   interviewer error..____ -9 | No answer/ |   interviewer error..____ -9 |
|  |   interviewer error..____ -9 |  |

| 4 | 5 | 6 |
|---|---|---|
| $7,200 or less...(56(   -1 | $7,200 or less...(58(   -1 | $7,200 or less...(60(   -1 |
| $7,201-9,300.........____ -2 | $7,201-11,000........____ -2 | $7,201-12,400.......____ -2 |
| $9,301-14,000.......____ -3 | $11,001-15,000......____ -3 | $12,401-15,000......____ -3 |
| $14,001-15,000......____ -4 | $15,001-16,500......____ -4 | $15,001-18,700......____ -4 |
| $15,001-25,000......____ -5 | $16,501-25,000......____ -5 | $18,701-25,000......____ -5 |
| $25,001-35,000......____ -6 | $25,001-35,000......____ -6 | $25,001-35,000......____ -6 |
| $35,001-50,000......____ -7 | $35,001-50,000......____ -7 | $35,001-50,000......____ -7 |
| Over $50,000.........____ -8 | Over $50,000.........____ -8 | Over $50,000.........____ -8 |
| Refused..........(57(   -7 | Refused..........(59(   -7 | Refused..........(61(   -7 |
| Not sure/don't know..____ -8 | Not sure/don't know..____ -8 | Not sure/don't know..____ -8 |
| No answer/ | No answer/ | No answer/ |
|   interviewer error..____ -9 |   interviewer error..____ -9 |   interviewer error..____ -9 |

| 7 | 8 | 9+ |
|---|---|---|
| $7,200 or less...(62(   -1 | $7,200 or less...(64(   -1 | $7,200 or less...(66(   -1 |
| $7,201-14,100.......____ -2 | $7,201-15,000........____ -2 | $7,201-15,000.......____ -2 |
| $14,101-15,000......____ -3 | $15,001-15,700......____ -3 | $15,001-18,700......____ -3 |
| $15,001-21,100......____ -4 | $15,701-23,500......____ -4 | $18,701-25,000......____ -4 |
| $21,101-25,000......____ -5 | $23,501-25,000......____ -5 | $25,001-28,000......____ -5 |
| $25,001-35,000......____ -6 | $25,001-35,000......____ -6 | $28,001-35,000......____ -6 |
| $35,001-50,000......____ -7 | $35,001-50,000......____ -7 | $35,001-50,000......____ -7 |
| Over $50,000.........____ -8 | Over $50,000.........____ -8 | Over $50,000.........____ -8 |
| Refused..........(63(   -7 | Refused..........(65(   -7 | Refused..........(67(   -7 |
| Not sure/don't know..____ -8 | Not sure/don't know..____ -8 | Not sure/don't know..____ -8 |
| No answer/ | No answer/ | No answer/ |
|   interviewer error..____ -9 |   interviewer error..____ -9 |   interviewer error..____ -9 |

|68Z|

-7-    CARD 01    824002

F7a.  For how many years have you (has s/he) lived in this community?
DO NOT READ LIST

| | |
|---|---|
| Less than 2 years........(69( | -1 |
| 2 to 5 years.................. | -2 |
| 6 to 10 years................ | -3 |
| 11 to 15 years............... | -4 |
| 16 to 20 years............... | -5 |
| More than 20 years........... | -6 |
| Refused...................... | -7 |
| Not sure/don't know.......... | -8 |
| No answer/interviewer error... | -9 |

F7b.  Do you live on a farm?  (IF IN DOUBT, ASK:  Did you sell $1,000 or more in agricultural products last year?)

| | |
|---|---|
| Yes......................(70( | -1 |
| No........................... | -2 |
| Refused...................... | -7 |
| Not sure/don't know.......... | -8 |
| No answer/interviewer error... | -9 |

INTERVIEWER:  CHECK SAMPLE CARD FOR ANY SPECIAL SAMPLING INSTRUCTIONS.  IF SPECIAL INSTRUCTION INDICATED ON CARD FOR THIS HOUSEHOLD, ASK APPROPRIATE QUESTION AT THIS POINT AND RECORD BELOW.  ALL CASES "1", "2", OR "3" SKIP TO Q.F8.

IF CLASS "4" OR "5", ASK Q.F7c
F7c.  Do you live in (READ NAME OF CITY), or not?

RECORD CITY NAME

CODE BELOW
| | | |
|---|---|---|
| Inside central city........(71( | -1 | |
| (4) Outside central city-SMSA....... | -2 | (SKIP TO Q.F8) |
| (5) Outside central city-Non-SMSA... | -3 | |

IF CLASS "6" OR "7" ASK Q.F7d
F7d.  What town, city, or village do you live in?

RECORD NAME

SAMPLING DEPARTMENT CODE BELOW
| | |
|---|---|
| Inside central city........(72( | -1 |
| Outside central city-SMSA....... | -2 |
| Outside central city-Non-SMSA... | -3 |

ASK EVERYONE    ASK Q.F8, Q.F9 FOR ADULT DESIGNATED RESPONDENT
F8.  Do you (does s/he) consider yourself (herself/himself) white, black, oriental, or what?

| | |
|---|---|
| White...................(73( | -1 |
| Black........................ | -2 |
| Oriental/Asian or Pacific Islander............ | -3 |
| American Indian or Alaskan native.............. | -4 |
| Refused...................... | -7 |
| Not sure/don't know.......... | -8 |
| No answer/interviewer error... | -9 |

F9.  Are you (is s/he) of Hispanic origin, or not?

| | |
|---|---|
| Hispanic origin...........(74( | -1 |
| Not of Hispanic origin........ | -2 |
| Refused...................... | -7 |
| Not sure/don't know.......... | -8 |
| No answer/interviewer error... | -9 |

F10: How many families use this telephone? By a family, we mean each group of people related by blood, marriage, or adoption.

```
1........................(75(____-1
2............................._____-2
3............................._____-3
4............................._____-4
5............................._____-5
6 or more....................._____-6
Refused......................._____-7
Not sure/don't know.........._____-8
No answer/interviewer error..._____-9
```

F11.    |INTERVIEWER:  CHECK SAMPLE CARD AND RECORD BELOW|
        FIRST INTERVIEW COMPLETED ON:

```
1st call......(76(____-1

2nd call........._____-2

3rd call........._____-3

4th call........._____-4

5th call........._____-5

6th call........._____-6

7th call........._____-7

8th call........._____-8
```

F12.   RECORD LANGUAGE OF INTERVIEW:

```
Spanish..................(77(____-1
English......................._____-2
Refused......................._____-7
Not sure/don't know.........._____-8
No answer/interviewer error..._____-9
```

|78-80Z|

ADULT INTERVIEW FROM GRID "A"

Begun Adult Interview:
Month: _____ / Date: _____ _____   Time: _____ : _____   o'clock  AM..(19(___ -1
       (11) (12)              (13) (14)        (15-16)  (17-18)              PM...... ___ -2

-1-      CARD 03         824002

1a.  If the Federal Government could spend more money on only one of the following
services, which one would you most like it spent on?

|READ FULL LIST BEFORE ACCEPTING ANY ANSWER -- SINGLE RECORD BELOW|

|  |  | Q.1a<br>First<br>Choice | Q.1b<br>Second<br>Choice |
|---|---|---|---|
| |START AT "X"| | |
| ( ) | Education.........................................(20(___ -1 | | (22(___ -1 |
| ( ) | Defense...............................................___ -2 | | ___ -2 |
| ( ) | Energy................................................___ -3 | | ___ -3 |
| ( ) | Welfare...............................................___ -4 | | ___ -4 |
| ( ) | Health care...........................................___ -5 | | ___ -5 |
| ( ) | Public transportation.................................___ -6 | | ___ -6 |
| ( ) | The environment.......................................___ -7 | | ___ -7 |
| ( ) | Unemployment..........................................___ -8 | | ___ -8 |
| ( ) | Housing...............................................___ -9 | | ___ -9 |
| ( ) | Social Security................................(21(___ -1 | | (23(___ -1 |
| | None of these (vol.)..................................___ -2 | | ___ -2 |
| | Refused...............................................___ -7 | | ___ -7 |
| | Not sure/don't know...................................___ -8 | | ___ -8 |
| | No answer/interviewer error..........................___ -9 | | ___ -9 |

1b.  And which service would be your second best choice for more money to be spent on?

|REREAD LIST IF NECESSARY -- SINGLE RECORD ABOVE|

1c.  Which of the following statements comes closest to expressing your overall view of
the American health care system?  |READ ALL THREE STATEMENTS BEFORE ACCEPTING AN ANSWER|
|SINGLE RECORD|

On the whole the health care system works pretty well
and only minor changes are necessary to make it work.........(24(___ -1

There are some good things in our health care system,
but fundamental changes are needed to make it work better........___ -2

The American health care system has so much wrong with it
that we need to completely rebuild it............................___ -3

Refused.........................................................___ -7

Not sure/don't know.............................................___ -8

No answer/interviewer error.....................................___ -9

|25-26Z|

IF PROXY INTERVIEW, SAY: Most of the questions in this interview will refer to (NAME OF ADULT SELECTED BY GRID "A").

2. Would you say your (her/his) health, in general, is excellent, good, fair, or poor?

            Excellent..........(27(____-1
            Good...................____-2
            Fair...................____-3
            Poor...................____-4
            Refused................____-7
            Not sure/don't know....____-8
            No answer/interviewer
               error..............____-9

3a. How many days altogether during the past year, that is, since (DATE ONE YEAR AGO) 1981, did you (s/he) stay in bed more than half of the day because of illness or injury? Include any days you (s/he) stayed in the hospital.

            _____Days  (28-30)
               (RECORD NUMBER)

            Refused..................(31(____-7
            Not sure/don't know..........____-8
            No answer/interviewer error...____-9

3b. Not counting the days in bed, how many days during the past year, that is, since (DATE ONE YEAR AGO) 1981, did you (s/he) have to cut down on the things you usually do (s/he usually does) for more than half of the day because of illness or injury? IF "NONE," RECORD "000"

            _____Days  (32-34)
               (RECORD NUMBER)

            Refused..................(35(____-7
            Not sure/don't know..........____-8
            No answer/interviewer error...____-9

IF PROXY INTERVIEW, SKIP TO Q.5a
4. In the past twelve months, that is, since (DATE ONE YEAR AGO) 1981, have you (READ EACH ITEM), or not?

|  | Yes, Have | No, Have Not | Re-fused | Not Sure/ Don't Know | No Answer/ Inter-viewer Error |
|---|---|---|---|---|---|
| a. Had a blood pressure reading.............(36( | -1 | -2 | -7 | -8 | -9 |
| b. Seen a dentist........................(37( | -1 | -2 | -7 | -8 | -9 |

ASK ITEMS c AND d OF WOMEN ONLY
| | | | | | |
|---|---|---|---|---|---|
| c. Had a Pap smear test for cancer.........(38( | -1 | -2 | -7 | -8 | -9 |
| d. Had a breast examination by a doctor.....(39( | -1 | -2 | -7 | -8 | -9 |

|ASK EVERYONE|

5a.  Is there one person or place in particular you (s/he) usually go(es) to when you are (s/he is) sick or (s/he) want(s) advice about your (her/his) health?

Yes, is person or place.......(40(___-1  (SKIP TO Q.6a)

No, is not........................____-2 ⎫
Refused..........................____-7 ⎬(ASK Q.5b)
Not sure/don't know..............____-8 ⎪
No answer/interviewer error.......____-9 ⎭

5b.  Many people do not have one particular place to get medical care.  How is it that you do (s/he does) not have a regular doctor or place to go?
|RECORD VERBATIM.  PROBE FOR COMPLETE ANSWER.|

_____    (41-43)

_____    (44-46)

_____    (47-49)

5c.  Is there a medical doctor or osteopath you (s/he) **might** go to if you (s/he) needed medical care?

Yes, there is............(50(___-1  (ASK Q.6a)

No, is not..................____-2 ⎫
Refused.....................____-7 ⎬(SKIP TO Q.7a)
Not sure/don't know..........____-8 ⎪
No answer/interviewer error...____-9 ⎭

6a.  Where do you (does s/he) usually go -- to a doctor's office, a clinic, a hospital, or some other place?

|PROBE WITH A, B, OR C BEFORE RECORDING.
A.  IF CLINIC:   Is it a private clinic; a hospital outpatient clinic; a company or union clinic; a school clinic; a neighborhood or government-sponsored clinic; or any other clinic not connected with a hospital?
|IF CAN'T SPECIFY, RECORD "CLINIC" UNDER "OTHER."|
B.  IF HOSPITAL:  Is it a hospital outpatient clinic or a hospital emergency room?
|IF CAN'T SPECIFY, RECORD "HOSPITAL" UNDER "OTHER."|
C.  IF SOME OTHER PLACE:  What type of place is it? |

Doctor's office or private clinic..........(51(___-1 ⎫
Company or union clinic........................____-2 ⎪
School clinic..................................____-3 ⎬(ASK Q.6b)
Neighborhood or government-sponsored clinic....____-4 ⎪
Hospital outpatient clinic.....................____-5 ⎪
Hospital emergency room........................____-6 ⎭

Health maintenance organization (HMO)..........____-7  (SKIP TO Q.6c)

Other place (SPECIFY)

_____..____-8  (ASK Q.6b)

Refused...................................(52(___-7 ⎫
Not sure/don't know...........................____-8 ⎬(SKIP TO Q.6c)
No answer/interviewer error...................____-9 ⎭

6b.  Is that place a health maintenance organization or HMO; that is, a place you go for all or most medical care, which is paid for by a fixed monthly or annual amount?

                    Is HMO..................(53(____ -1

                    Isn't HMO...................____ -2
                    Refused.....................____ -7
                    Not sure/don't know.........____ -8
                    No answer/interviewer error...____ -9

6c.  Is there one particular doctor you (s/he) usually see(s) when you (s/he) go(es) there?

                    Yes, is..................(54(____ -1  (ASK Q.6d)

                    No, is not..................____ -2 ⎫
                    Refused.....................____ -7 ⎬ (SKIP TO Q.6e)
                    Not sure/don't know.........____ -8 ⎪
                    No answer/interviewer error...____ -9 ⎭

6d.  What is his or her name?

                    _____
                              (RECORD NAME)

INTERVIEWER CODE
Yes, doctor named..........................(55(____ -1
No, doctor not named..........................____ -2
Refused.......................................____ -7
Not sure/don't know...........................____ -8
No answer/interviewer error...................____ -9

6e.  How long have you (has s/he) been going to (PLACE MENTIONED IN Q.6a)?
DO NOT READ LIST

                    Less than 1 year.........(56(____ -1
                    1 year but less than 2 years..____ -2
                    2 years.....................____ -3
                    3 years.....................____ -4
                    4 years.....................____ -5
                    5 years.....................____ -6
                    6 years or more (SPECIFY:
                      WRITE IN YEARS)

                    _____ ____ (57-58)
                    Refused..................(59.____ -7
                    Not sure/don't know.........____ -8
                    No answer/interviewer error...____ -9

ASK EVERYONE
7a.  What was the month and year of your (her/his) most recent medical visit -- when you (s/he) actually saw a doctor in an office or at a clinic?

                    Month:_____  Year:_____

IF PRIOR TO 1981, RECORD YEAR ONLY  DO NOT PROBE FOR MONTH

                    Within last 12 months.......(60(____ -1  (ASK Q.7b)

                    Longer ago (SPECIFY)

                    _____ (61-62)
                    RECORD NUMBER OF YEARS              (SKIP TO Q.8)
                    Refused..................(63(____ -7
                    Not sure/don't know.........____ -8
                    No answer/interviewer error.....____ -9

7b. To what type of place did you (s/he) go for this last visit -- did you (s/he) go to a doctor's office, a clinic, a hospital, or some other place?

```
PROBE WITH A, B, OR C BEFORE RECORDING.
A.  IF CLINIC:   Was it a private clinic; a hospital outpatient clinic; a company or
                 union clinic; a school clinic; a neighborhood or government-sponsored
                 clinic; or any other clinic not connected with a hospital?
                 IF CAN'T SPECIFY, RECORD "CLINIC" UNDER "OTHER."

B.  IF HOSPITAL:  Was it a hospital outpatient clinic or a hospital emergency room?
                  IF CAN'T SPECIFY, RECORD "HOSPITAL" UNDER "OTHER."

C.  IF SOME OTHER PLACE:  What type of place was it?
```

Doctor's office or private clinic.........(64(____-1 ⎞
Company or union clinic.........................____-2 ⎟
School clinic.......................................____-3 ⎬(ASK Q.7c)
Neighborhood or government-sponsored clinic....____-4 ⎟
Hospital outpatient clinic.......................____-5 ⎟
Hospital emergency room..........................____-6 ⎠

Health maintenance organization (HMO)..........____-7  (SKIP TO Q.7d)

Other place (SPECIFY)

_____..____-8  (ASK Q.7c)

Refused......................................(65(____-7 ⎞
Not sure/don't know...........................____-8 ⎬(SKIP TO Q.7d)
No answer/interviewer error...................____-9 ⎠

7c. Was that place a health maintenance organization or HMO (that is, a place you go for all or most medical care, which is paid for by a fixed monthly or annual amount)?

Was HMO...................(66(____-1
Wasn't HMO......................____-2
Refused.........................____-7
Not sure/don't know...........____-8
No answer/interviewer error...____-9

    ⎡67-80Z⎤

7d. Is this the place you (s/he) usually go(es) to for care, or not?

Yes, is place usually go........(11(____-1  (SKIP TO Q.7f)

No, isn't place usually go...........____-2  (ASK Q.7e)

Refused.............................____-7 ⎞
Not sure/don't know.................____-8 ⎬(SKIP TO Q.7f)
No answer/interviewer error.........____-9 ⎠

-6-    CARD 04    824002

7e. Why didn't you (s/he) go to the place you (s/he) usually go(es) for medical care the last time you were (s/he was) sick? |DO NOT READ LIST, MULTIPLE RECORD|

Couldn't get an appointment............(12(____-1
It cost too much for a visit..........(13(____-1
Had no way to get there...............(14(____-1
It was an emergency...................(15(____-1
Need a specialist/specific service.....(16(____-1
Referred by usual source..............(17(____-1
Other (SPECIFY)

_____(18(____-1
Refused.............................(19(____-1
Not sure/don't know.......................____-8
No answer/interviewer error.................____-9

7f. How long did you (s/he) have to wait to see the doctor once you (s/he) got there? |RECORD AND CIRCLE HOURS OR MINUTES|

Number:_____    Hours
                                    Minutes    ‾(20)‾ ‾(21)‾ ‾(22)‾

Refused...................(23(____-7
Not sure/don't know...........____-8
No answer/interviewer error...____-9

|IF PROXY INTERVIEW, SKIP TO Q.10|
7g. During your last visit for medical care, were you completely satisfied, somewhat satisfied, or not at all satisfied with (READ EACH ITEM)?

| |START AT "X"| | Completely Satisfied | Somewhat Satisfied | Not At All Satis- fied | Re- fused | Not Sure/ Don't Know | No Answer/ Inter- viewer Error |
|---|---|---|---|---|---|---|---|
| ( ) a. | The amount of time it took you to get there......(24( | ____-1 | ____-2 | ____-3 | ____-7 | ____-8 | ____-9 |
| ( ) b. | The amount of time you had to wait to see the doctor, once there................(25( | ____-1 | ____-2 | ____-3 | ____-7 | ____-8 | ____-9 |
| ( ) c. | The amount of time the doctor spent with you......(26( | ____-1 | ____-2 | ____-3 | ____-7 | ____-8 | ____-9 |
| ( ) d. | The information given to you about what was wrong with you, or about what was being done for you.....(27( | ____-1 | ____-2 | ____-3 | ____-7 | ____-8 | ____-9 |
| ( ) e. | The out-of-pocket cost for the medical care received, that is, the cost not paid by insurance...............(28( | ____-1 | ____-2 | ____-3 | ____-7 | ____-8 | ____-9 |
| ( ) f. | The quality of the care you felt was provided at that visit....................(29( | ____-1 | ____-2 | ____-3 | ____-7 | ____-8 | ____-9 |
| |ASK ITEM "g" LAST| | | | | | | |
| g. | This visit to the doctor, overall...................(30( | ____-1 | ____-2 | ____-3 | ____-7 | ____-8 | ____-9 |

|SKIP TO Q.10|

8. Did you (s/he) <u>see</u> or <u>talk</u> to a doctor any time during the past twelve months, that is since (DATE ONE YEAR AGO) 1981? This includes visits to the doctor and any visit to a nurse or other medical person on the doctor's staff, instead of the doctor.

> Yes, saw or talked to......(31(    -1  (SKIP TO Q.10)
>
> No, didn't see or talk to......_____-2  (ASK Q.9)
>
> Refused........................_____-7 ⎫
> Not sure/don't know............_____-8 ⎬(SKIP TO Q.10)
> No answer/interviewer error...._____-9 ⎭

9. Why haven't you (hasn't s/he) seen or spoken with a doctor in the last year?
⌐DO NOT READ LIST -- MULTIPLE RECORD⌐

> Wasn't sick/didn't need one..................(32(   -1
> Didn't know a doctor or clinic to go to......(33(   -1
> Couldn't afford to go/didn't have insurance..(34(   -1
> Doesn't like doctors.........................(35(   -1
> Other (SPECIFY)
>
> _____ (36(   -1
> Refused......................................(37(   -7
> Not sure/don't know..............................._____-8
> No answer/interviewer error......................._____-9

⌐SKIP TO Q.11a⌐

10. How many of each of the following kinds of visits did you (s/he) have with a doctor or doctor's assistant during the past twelve months, that is, since (DATE ONE YEAR AGO) 1981?

⌐READ EACH ITEM AND RECORD NUMBER OF VISITS. IF "NOT SURE," RECORD "999."
IF "NONE," RECORD "000."

Number of Visits

House calls by a doctor or doctor's assistant............._____
                                                                (38-39-40)

Visits to a doctor's office or private clinic............._____
                                                                 (41-42-43)

Visits to a company or union clinic......................._____
                                                                 (44-45-46)

Visits to a school clinic................................._____
                                                                 (47-48-49)

Visits to a neighborhood or government-sponsored clinic..._____
                                                              (50-51-52)

Visits to a hospital outpatient clinic..................._____
                                                                 (53-54-55)

Visits to a hospital emergency room......................._____
                                                              (56-57-58)

Visits to any other place for medical care, other than when you may have been a patient overnight in a hospital (SPECIFY)

_____...._____
             (62)                                              (59-60-61)

|ASK EVERYONE|
11a. Did you (s/he) talk on the telephone to a doctor or doctor's assistant for
prescriptions or medical advice any time during the past twelve months, that is, since
(DATE ONE YEAR AGO) 1981?

Yes, did talk............(63(___-1  (ASK Q.11b)

No, didn't talk..............___-2 ⎫
Refused.....................___-7 ⎬ (SKIP TO Q.12)
Not sure/don't know..........___-8 ⎪
No answer/interviewer error...___-9 ⎭

11b.  How many times did you (s/he) talk on the telephone to a doctor or doctor's
assistant for prescriptions or medical advice?

_____  (64-65)
(RECORD NUMBER)
Refused...................(66(___-7
Not sure/don't know..........___-8
No answer/interviewer error...___-9

12.  Have you (has s/he) personally had a medical emergency anytime in the last year --
since (DATE ONE YEAR AGO) 1981 -- or not?

Yes, have had medical emergency........(67(___-1  (ASK Q.13a)

No, have not had medical emergency..........___-2 ⎫
Refused....................................___-7 ⎬ (SKIP TO Q.17a)
Not sure/don't know........................___-8 ⎪
No answer/interviewer error................___-9 ⎭

13a.  To what type of place did you (s/he) go for emergency medical care -- to a
doctor's office, a clinic, a hospital, or some other place?
|IF MORE THAN ONE EPISODE, PROBE FOR MOST RECENT|

---

PROBE WITH A, B, OR C BEFORE RECORDING.
A.  IF CLINIC:  Was it a private clinic; a hospital outpatient clinic; a company or
                union clinic; a school clinic; a neighborhood or government-sponsored
                clinic; or any other clinic not connected with a hospital?
                |IF CAN'T SPECIFY, RECORD "CLINIC" UNDER "OTHER."|

B.  IF HOSPITAL:  Was it a hospital outpatient clinic or a hospital emergency room?
                  |IF CAN'T SPECIFY, RECORD "HOSPITAL" UNDER "OTHER."|

C.  IF SOME OTHER PLACE:  What type of place was it?

---

Doctor's office or private clinic..........(68(___-1 ⎫
Company or union clinic.......................___-2 ⎪
School clinic.................................___-3 ⎬ (ASK Q.13b)
Neighborhood or government-sponsored clinic....___-4 ⎪
Hospital outpatient clinic....................___-5 ⎪
Hospital emergency room.......................___-6 ⎭

Health maintenance organization (HMO)..........___-7  (SKIP TO Q.14)

Other place (SPECIFY)

_____ ..___-8  (ASK Q.13b)

Didn't go anywhere............................___-9  (SKIP TO Q.17a)

Refused....................................(69(___-7 ⎫
Not sure/don't know...........................___-8 ⎬ (SKIP TO Q.14)
No answer/interviewer error...................___-9 ⎭

13b.  Was that place a health maintenance organization or HMO (that is, a place you go for all or most medical care, which is paid for by a fixed monthly or annual amount)?

```
                    Was  HMO...................(11(____ -1
                    Wasn't HMO....................____ -2
                    Refused.......................____ -7
                    Not sure/don't know...........____ -8
                    No answer/interviewer error...____ -9
```

14.  What was the health problem or condition at that time?

_____     (12-15)

_____     (16-19)

_____     (20-23)

15a.  Did you (s/he) have any problems in getting there, or not?

```
                    Yes, had problems..........(24(____ -1  (ASK Q.15b)

                    No, didn't have problems........____ -2 ⟍
                    Refused.........................____ -7  ⟩(SKIP TO Q.16)
                    Not sure/don't know.............____ -8  /
                    No answer/interviewer error.....____ -9 ⟋
```

15b.  What were the problems in getting there?  What else?

_____     (25-26)

_____     (27-28)

_____     (29-30)

| IF PROXY INTERVIEW, SKIP TO Q.17a |

16.  Thinking about that experience with emergency care, were you completely satisfied, somewhat satisfied, or not at all satisfied with (READ EACH ITEM)?

| | | | Completely Satisfied | Somewhat Satisfied | Not At All Satis- fied | Re- fused | Not Sure/ Don't Know | No Answer/ Inter- viewer Error |
|---|---|---|---|---|---|---|---|---|
| START AT "X" | | | | | | | | |
| ( ) | a. | The amount of time it took you to get there......(31( | -1 | -2 | -3 | -7 | -8 | -9 |
| ( ) | b. | The amount of time you had to wait to see the doctor, once there.................(32( | -1 | -2 | -3 | -7 | -8 | -9 |
| ( ) | c. | The amount of time the doctor spent with you......(33( | -1 | -2 | -3 | -7 | -8 | -9 |
| ( ) | d. | The information given to you about what was wrong with you or about what was being done for you.........(34( | -1 | -2 | -3 | -7 | -8 | -9 |
| ( ) | e. | The out-of-pocket cost of the medical care you received, that is, the cost not paid by insurance......(35( | -1 | -2 | -3 | -7 | -8 | -9 |
| ( ) | f. | The quality of the care you felt was provided at that visit................(36( | -1 | -2 | -3 | -7 | -8 | -9 |

| ASK ITEM "g" LAST |

| | g. | This visit to the doctor, overall...................(37( | -1 | -2 | -3 | -7 | -8 | -9 |

| ASK EVERYONE |

17a.  Have you (has s/he) been a patient overnight in a hospital during the past twelve months, since (DATE ONE YEAR AGO) 1981?

```
            Yes, has been a patient.........(38(    -1  (ASK Q.17b)

            No, has not been a patient...........    -2
            Refused..............................    -7  } (SKIP TO Q.22)
            Not sure/don't know..................    -8
            No answer/interviewer error..........    -9
```

17b.  How many times were you (was s/he) admitted to a hospital since (DATE ONE YEAR AGO) 1981?

```
            _____ Times  (39-41)
                (RECORD NUMBER)
            Refused...................(42(    -7
            Not sure/don't know...........    -8
            No answer/interviewer error...    -9
```

17c.  Altogether, how many nights did you (s/he) stay in a hospital during that period, that is since (DATE ONE YEAR AGO) 1981?

```
            _____ Nights  (43-45)
                (RECORD NUMBER)
            Refused...................(46(    -7
            Not sure/don't know...........    -8
            No answer/interviewer error...    -9
```

-11-    CARD 05    824002

18. The last time you were in the hospital overnight were you completely satisfied, somewhat satisfied, or not at all satisfied with (READ EACH ITEM)?

| START AT "X" | Completely Satisfied | Somewhat Satisfied | Not At All Satisfied | Refused | Not Sure/ Don't Know | No Answer/ Interviewer Error |
|---|---|---|---|---|---|---|
| (  ) a. The availability of doctors whenever they were needed....(47( | -1 | -2 | -3 | -7 | -8 | -9 |
| (  ) b. The availability of nurses whenever they were needed....(48( | -1 | -2 | -3 | -7 | -8 | -9 |
| (  ) c. The out-of-pocket cost to you of the care received -- that is, the cost not paid by insurance.......(49( | -1 | -2 | -3 | -7 | -8 | -9 |
| (  ) d. The information given to you about what was wrong with you or about what was being done for you............(50( | -1 | -2 | -3 | -7 | -8 | -9 |
| (  ) e. The quality of the care received from doctors in the hospital...........(51( | -1 | -2 | -3 | -7 | -8 | -9 |
| ASK ITEM "f" LAST (  ) f. The overall quality of the care you felt you got at the hospital...........(52( | -1 | -2 | -3 | -7 | -8 | -9 |

IF PROXY INTERVIEW, SAY:    Thinking about the last time (s/he) was in the hospital overnight...

19. What was the health problem or condition leading to that hospital stay?

_____    (53-56)

_____    (57-60)

_____    (61-64)

-12-        CARD 05            824002

|IF PROXY INTERVIEW, SKIP TO Q.21|

20a.  Was any kind of surgery performed during that hospital stay, or not?

Yes, some kind of surgery was performed...(65(____-1  (ASK Q.20b)

No, no surgery was performed...................____-2 ⎫
Refused........................................____-7 ⎬ (SKIP TO Q.21)
Not sure/don't know............................____-8 ⎪
No answer/interviewer error....................____-9 ⎭

20b.  What kind of operation was this?

_____  (66-67)

_____  (68-69)

_____  (70-71)

21.  About how much did you or your family pay for the hospital bills for that stay?
Don't count any bills that insurance may have paid or that you think that insurance will
pay.  |PROBE FOR BEST ESTIMATE, DO NOT READ LIST|

$0/nothing................(72(____-1
$1-100.......................____-2
$101-200.....................____-3
$201-400.....................____-4
$401-600.....................____-5
$601-1,000...................____-6
$1,001-2,000.................____-7
Over $2,000..................____-8
Refused..................(73(____-7
Not sure/don't know..........____-8
No answer/interviewer error...____-9

|74-80Z|

-13-    CARD 06    824002

22. Now I'd like to talk about the different kinds of health plans or health insurance that people have, including those provided by the government. As I read each of the following health plans, please tell me whether you are (s/he is) covered by it.
|READ EACH ITEM|

| | Yes, Covered | No, Not Covered | Refused | Not Sure/ Don't Know | No Answer/ Inter- viewer Error |
|---|---|---|---|---|---|
| Health insurance through work or union....(11( | -1 | -2 | -7 | -8 | -9 |
| Health insurance through some other group.................................(12( | -1 | -2 | -7 | -8 | -9 |
| Health insurance bought directly by yourself (herself/himself) or your (her/his) family........................(13( | -1 | -2 | -7 | -8 | -9 |
| Medicare A, that pays hospital bills for people aged 65 and over and for some disabled people................ ...(14( | -1 | -2 | -7 | -8 | -9 |
| Medicare B, that pays doctor's bills for people aged 65 and over and for some disabled people....................(15( | -1 | -2 | -7 | -8 | -9 |
| Medicaid or Public Aid...................(16( | -1 | -2 | -7 | -8 | -9 |
| Prepaid group practice or an HMO (that is, a place you go for all or most medical care which is paid for by a fixed monthly or annual amount) (USE PROBE BELOW)......(17( | -1 | -2 | -7 | -8 | -9 |
| Another clinic or health care center where you (s/he) can get care at no cost or at reduced rates.................(18( | -1 | -2 | -7 | -8 | -9 |
| Any other place? (SPECIFY) (IF RESPONDENT SAYS "BLUE CROSS" OR "BLUE SHIELD" OR NAMES A SPECIFIC INSURANCE COMPANY, USE PROBE BELOW AND DO NOT RECORD HERE.) _____ (20) ...(19( | -1 | -2 | -7 | -8 | -9 |

|PROBE: Was it purchased through work or a union, through some other group, bought directly by yourself (herself/himself), or the family, or purchased some other way? |RECORD ABOVE||

|IF "NO" OR "NOT SURE" FOR ALL ITEMS IN Q.22, SKIP TO Q.24.|
23. Does your (her/his) health insurance coverage pay for part, all, or none of the cost of (READ EACH ITEM)?

| |START AT "X"| | Part | All | None | Refused | Not Sure/ Don't Know | No Answer/ Inter- viewer Error |
|---|---|---|---|---|---|---|---|
| ( ) | a. Visits to the doctor's office...................(21( | -1 | -2 | -3 | -7 | -8 | -9 |
| ( ) | b. Hospital expenses........(22( | -1 | -2 | -3 | -7 | -8 | -9 |
| ( ) | c. Surgical expenses.......(23( | -1 | -2 | -3 | -7 | -8 | -9 |
| ( ) | d. Prescribed medicine taken outside of the hospital..(24( | -1 | -2 | -3 | -7 | -8 | -9 |

-14-        CARD 06             824002

24.  Has your (her/his) health coverage, that is the benefits provided by your (her/his) health insurance, changed in the last year since (DATE ONE YEAR AGO) 1981, or not?

Yes changed...............(25(____-1  (ASK Q.25a)

No, hasn't changed...........____-2
Refused.......................____-7   (SKIP TO Q.27)
Not sure/don't know..........____-8
No answer/interviewer error...____-9


25a.  How has your health coverage changed in the last year?

_____                (26-27)

_____                (28-29)

_____                (30-31)


25b.  Why has your health coverage or health insurance changed in the last year?

|DO NOT READ LIST, SINGLE RECORD|

Changed jobs....................(32(____-1
Lost job...........................____-2
Changed insurer.....................____-3
Voluntarily increased coverage......____-4
Voluntarily decreased coverage......____-5
Other (SPECIFY)

_____.......____-6
Refused...........................____-7
Not sure/don't know................____-8
No answer/interviewer error........____-9


26.  Because of the change in your (her/his) health insurance, in the past year, have you (has s/he) (READ EACH ITEM), or not?

| |START AT "X"| | Yes, Have | No, Haven't | Refused | Not Sure/ Don't Know | No Answer/ Inter- viewer Error |
|---|---|---|---|---|---|
| ( )  a.  Been unable to get some kind of health care............(33( | ____-1 | ____-2 | ____-7 | ____-8 | ____-9 |
| ( )  b.  Changed your (her/his) doctor or the place where you (s/he) usually go(es) for your (her/his) care health ...................,(34( | ____-1 | ____-2 | ____-7 | ____-8 | ____-9 |
| ( )  c.  Put off getting any kind of health care....................(35( | ____-1 | ____-2 | ____-7 | ____-8 | ____-9 |

27.  In the last year have you (has s/he) gotten any medical care or health care services free because you were (s/he was) not covered by insurance and could not afford to pay for it, or not?

Obtained free care........(36(____-1
Not obtained free care........____-2
Refused.......................____-7
Not sure/don't know...........____-8
No answer/interviewer error...____-9

28a. The next questions apply to you and all the other members of your family who live with you. Was there any time in the last year -- since (DATE ONE YEAR AGO) 1981 -- that you felt you or a member of your family living with you needed medical help but did not get it for some reason?

Yes, was a time..........(37(____-1  (ASK Q.28b)

No, wasn't....................____-2 ⎫
Refused.......................____-7 ⎬(SKIP TO Q.31)
Not sure/don't know...........____-8 ⎪
No answer/interviewer error...____-9 ⎭

28b. Which members of your family needed medical help but did not get it?
|MULTIPLE RECORD|

|  | Q.28b | Q.28c Person With Most Recent Episode |
|---|---|---|
| Self/proxy....................... | ____(38-39) | ____(48-49) |
| _____ | ____(40-41) | ____(50-51) |
| _____ | ____(42-43) | ____(52-53) |
| _____ | ____(44-45) | ____(54-55) |
| _____ | ____(46-47) | ____(56-57) |

INTERVIEWER: IF MORE THAN ONE IN Q.28b, ASK: "Who had the most recent experience?" AND "X" APPROPRIATE LINE IN Q.28c ABOVE.

28d. Thinking about the most recent time this happened, did anyone in your family try to get medical help?

Yes, someone tried.......(58(____-1  (ASK Q.28e)

No, no one tried..............____-2  (SKIP TO Q.29)

Refused.......................____-7 ⎫
Not sure/don't know...........____-8 ⎬(SKIP TO Q.30)
No answer/interviewer error...____-9 ⎭

28e. What was the main reason that your family was not able to get the medical help needed in this situation?
|DO NOT READ LIST, SINGLE RECORD|

a. Could not get an appointment............(59(____-1
b. Did not know a good doctor or
   clinic to go to.............................____-2
c. It cost too much............................____-3
d. Could not get off work......................____-4
e. Couldn't find anyone to take care
   of the children.............................____-5
f. Would have had to wait too long
   in the doctor's office or clinic............____-6
g. There was no easy way to get to the
   doctor's office or clinic...................____-7
h. Couldn't find a doctor who speaks
   your language...............................____-8
i. Not covered by insurance....................____-9
j. Too nervous or afraid...................(60(____-1
k. Other (SPECIFY)
   _____ ..____-2
Refused..........................................____-7
Not sure/don't know..............................____-8
No answer/interviewer error......................____-9

|SKIP TO Q.30|

-16-        CARD 06                    824002

29. What was the <u>main</u> reason no one in your family tried to see a doctor about this situation?
<u>DO NOT READ LIST, SINGLE RECORD</u>

    a. Could not get an appointment............(61(____-1
    b. Did not know a good doctor or
       clinic to go to.............................____-2
    c. It cost too much............................____-3
    d. Could not get off work.....................____-4
    e. Couldn't find anyone to take care
       of the children............................____-5
    f. Would have had to wait too long
       in the doctor's office or clinic............____-6
    g. There was no easy way to get to the
       doctor's office or clinic...................____-7
    h. Couldn't find a doctor who speaks
       your language..............................____-8
    i. Not covered by insurance....................____-9
    j. Too nervous or afraid..................(62(____-1
    k. Condition not serious enough................____-2
    l. Other (SPECIFY)

    _____..____-3
    Refused.........................................____-7
    Not sure/don't know.............................____-8
    No answer/interviewer error.....................____-9

30. What was the health problem or condition at that time?

_____ (63-66)

_____ (67-70)

_____ (71-74)

<u>ASK EVERYONE</u>
31. During the last year -- since (DATE ONE YEAR AGO) 1981 -- have you or has any member of your family living with you been refused health care because you didn't have insurance or you couldn't pay, or for any other reason?

    Yes, refused for financial reason...(75(____-1
    No, not refused.........................____-2
    Refused for other reason (SPECIFY)

    _____..____-3
    Refused.................................____-7
    Not sure/don't know.....................____-8
    No answer/interviewer error.............____-9

76-80Z

-17-    CARD 07    824002

|ASK Q.32a AND Q.32b CONSECUTIVELY FOR EACH ITEM|
32a.  I'm going to read you a list of different health care services.  For each one,
please tell me if it is a service that you or someone in your family living with you
tried to get in the last year, but could not get for some reason.

|READ EACH ITEM, RECORD BELOW|

|ASK Q.32b FOR EACH "TRIED TO GET AND COULD NOT" IN Q.32a|
32b.  Who in your family needed (SERVICE IN Q.32a)?
|MULTIPLE RECORD, IF NECESSARY, BELOW|

|  |  | Q.32a |  |  |  |  |
|---|---|---|---|---|---|---|
|  |  | Tried To Get But Could Not | No (Didn't Try/Tried And Got) | Refused | Not Sure/ Don't Know | No Answer/ Inter- viewer Error | Q.32b Who Needed |
| a. | Emergency medical care........(11( | -1 | -2 | -7 | -8 | -9 | (21-22) (23-24) (25-26) |
| b. | An overnight hospital stay.......(12( | -1 | -2 | -7 | -8 | -9 | (27-28) (29-30) (31-32) |
| c. | Services at home, such as a visiting nurse, or doctor....(13( | -1 | -2 | -7 | -8 | -9 | (33-34) (35-36) (37-38) |
| d. | Mental health services or psychiatric counseling.........(14( | -1 | -2 | -7 | -8 | -9 | (39-40) (41-42) (43-44) |
| e. | Treatment of drug or drinking problem....(15( | -1 | -2 | -7 | -8 | -9 | (45-46) (47-48) (49-50) |
| f. | Family planning services or birth control............(16( | -1 | -2 | -7 | -8 | -9 | (51-52) (53-54) (55-56) |
| g. | Services of a pharmacy or drugstore at night and on weekends.....(17( | -1 | -2 | -7 | -8 | -9 | (57-58) (59-60) (61-62) |
| h. | Nursing home facilities..........(18( | -1 | -2 | -7 | -8 | -9 | (63-64) (65-66) (67-68) |

|ASK ITEM "i" ONLY IF CHILDREN IN FAMILY|

| i. | Services of a pediatrician or children's doctor...(19( | -1 | -2 | -7 | -8 | -9 | (69-70) (71-72) (73-74) |

|ASK ITEM "j" ONLY IF FEMALE IN FAMILY|

| j. | Care for a pregnant family member.......(20( | -1 | -2 | -7 | -8 | -9 | (75-76) (77-78) (79-80) |

33.  In the last twelve months, has it been easier or more difficult for you and your family to get the medical help you need, or hasn't it changed in the last year?

    Easier...................(11(    -1  (SKIP TO Q.35)

    More difficult...............___-2  (ASK Q.34)

    Hasn't changed................___-3 ⎫
    Refused......................___-7 ⎬(SKIP TO Q.35)
    Not sure/don't know..........___-8 ⎪
    No answer/interviewer error...___-9 ⎭

34.  How is it more difficult now for you and your family to get the medical help you need?  What else?

_____  (12-13)

_____  (14-15)

_____  (16-17)

|ASK EVERYONE|
35.  Including yourself, is there anyone in your family living with you who has a serious illness, is chronically sick, or who needs medical treatment or hospitalization on a regular basis?

    Yes, there is..........(18(    -1  (ASK Q.36)

    No, is not.................___-2 ⎫
    Refused....................___-7 ⎬(SKIP TO INSTRUCTIONS FOLLOWING Q.41)
    Not sure/don't know........___-8 ⎪
    No answer/interviewer error.___-9 ⎭

36.  How many people in your family are there who have a serious illness, are chronically sick, or who need medical treatment or hospitalization fairly often?

    One.....................(19(    -1
    Two..........................___-2
    Three or more................___-3
    Refused......................___-7
    Not sure/don't know..........___-8
    No answer/interviewer error...___-9

37a.  Which member(s) of your family is that (are those)?   |RECORD NAMES BELOW|

|   | Q.37a<br>Name or Other Description |   | Q.37b<br>Condition |
|---|---|---|---|
| 1. | _____ ___(20-21) | | _____ (30-33) |
| 2. | _____ ___(22-23) | | _____ (34-37) |
| 3. | _____ ___(24-25) | | _____ (38-41) |
| 4. | _____ ___(26-27) | | _____ (42-45) |
| 5. | _____ ___(28-29) | | _____ (46-49) |

37b.  What is (READ EACH NAME IN Q.37a)'s illness or condition?   |RECORD ABOVE|

38.  Does that person (do any of those people) need to have someone present in the house at all times, or not?

    Yes, need(s).............(50(    -1
    No, do(es) not need...........___-2
    Refused......................___-7
    Not sure/don't know..........___-8
    No answer/interviewer error...___-9

-19-        CARD 08              824002

39a.  Has anyone in the family made a major change in job, housing, or living arrangements because of that person's illness (those persons' illnesses)?

Yes, has made change......(51(___-1  (ASK Q.39b)

No, has not made change.......___-2
Refused.......................___-7  (SKIP TO Q.40)
Not sure/don't know..........___-8
No answer/interviewer error...___-9

39b.  What was the nature of the change?
[PROBE FOR DETAILS AND ADDITIONAL MAJOR CHANGES]

_____  (52-53)

_____  (54-55)

_____  (56-57)

40.  During the past twelve months, has your family looked for but been unable to get (READ EACH ITEM), or not?

| [START AT "X"] | Looked For But Couldn't Get | Did Not Look For/ Looked For And Got | Refused | Not Sure/ Don't Know | No Answer/ Interviewer Error |
|---|---|---|---|---|---|
| ( )  a.  A physical therapist to visit your home.................(58( | -1 | -2 | -7 | -8 | -9 |
| ( )  b.  A mental health counselor or social worker to visit your home........................(59( | -1 | -2 | -7 | -8 | -9 |
| ( )  c.  A housekeeper.....................(60( | -1 | -2 | -7 | -8 | -9 |
| ( )  d.  A nurse visiting your home........(61( | -1 | -2 | -7 | -8 | -9 |
| ( )  e.  Meals on wheels at home...........(62( | -1 | -2 | -7 | -8 | -9 |
| ( )  f.  Transportation to the doctor or hospital.......................(63( | -1 | -2 | -7 | -8 | -9 |
| ( )  g.  Medical appliances or equipment in your home......................(64( | -1 | -2 | -7 | -8 | -9 |
| ( )  h.  Nursing home or any other long term care outside of the home......(65( | -1 | -2 | -7 | -8 | -9 |
| ( )  i.  Home dental care..................(66( | -1 | -2 | -7 | -8 | -9 |

41.  How serious a financial problem has illness been to your family in the last year -- has it been a major problem, a minor problem, or has it been no financial problem at all?

Major problem............(67(___-1
Minor problem.................___-2
No problem at all.......•......___-3
Refused......................___-7
Not sure/don't know..........___-8
No answer/interviewer error...___-9

[INTERVIEWER NOTE:

IF CHILD PROXY AND FACTUALS ALREADY COMPLETED, THANK AND TERMINATE.

IF NO CHILDREN IN HOUSEHOLD, GO TO FACTUALS ATTACHED TO SCREEN FOR THIS HOUSEHOLD.

IF CHILDREN IN HOUSEHOLD AND SAME RESPONDENT SELECTED BY GRIDS A AND B, CONTINUE WITH CHILD PROXY INTERVIEW AND THEN ASK FACTUALS ATTACHED TO SCREEN FOR THIS HOUSEHOLD.

IF CHILDREN IN HOUSEHOLD AND DIFFERENT RESPONDENTS SELECTED BY GRIDS A AND B, ASK FACTUALS ATTACHED TO SCREEN FOR THIS HOUSEHOLD NEXT; THEN ASK TO SPEAK WITH SELECTED ADULT FOR CHILD PROXY.]

Time at this Point:  _____ : _____  o'clock  AM..(72(___-1
                     (68-69)  (70-71)            PM......___-2              [73-80Z]

CHILD PROXY INTERVIEW FROM GRID "B"

NAME OF CHILD SELECTED BY GRID "B" _____

(WRITE IN)

Begun Child Proxy Interview:
Month: _____ / Date: _____  Time: _____ : _____ o'clock AM..(19( ___ -1
   $\overline{(11)}$ $\overline{(12)}$    $\overline{(13)}$ $\overline{(14)}$    $\overline{(15-16)}$  $\overline{(17-18)}$         PM..... ___ -2

                              -20-      CARD 09        824002

42. All of these questions are going to be about (NAME OF CHILD SELECTED BY GRID "B").
Would you say (her/his) health, in general, is excellent, good, fair, or poor?

               Excellent.................(27( ___ -1
               Good......................... ___ -2          |20-26Z|
               Fair......................... ___ -3
               Poor......................... ___ -4
               Refused...................... ___ -7
               Not sure/don't know.......... ___ -8
               No answer/interviewer error... ___ -9

43a. How many days altogether during the past year, that is, since (DATE ONE YEAR AGO)
1981, did (s/he) stay in bed more than half of the day because of illness or injury?
Include any days (s/he) stayed in the hospital.

               _____ Days   (28-30)
               (RECORD NUMBER)

               Refused...................(31( ___ -7
               Not sure/don't know.......... ___ -8
               No answer/interviewer error... ___ -9

43b. Not counting the days in bed, how many days during the past year, that is, since
(DATE ONE YEAR AGO) 1981, did (s/he) have to cut down on the things (s/he) usually does
for more than half of the day because of illness or injury?
|IF "NONE," RECORD "000"|

               _____ Days   (32-34)
               (RECORD NUMBER)

               Refused...................(35( ___ -7
               Not sure/don't know.......... ___ -8       |36-39Z|
               No answer/interviewer error... ___ -9

44a. Is there one person or place in particular (s/he) usually goes to when (s/he) is
sick or when you want advice about (her/his) health?

        Yes, is person or place.......(40( ___ -1  (SKIP TO Q.45a)

        No................................ ___ -2 )
        Refused........................... ___ -7  \ (ASK Q.44b)
        Not sure/don't know............... ___ -8  /
        No answer/interviewer error....... ___ -9 )

   44b. Many people do not have one particular place to get medical care. How is it
   that (s/he) does not have a regular doctor or place to go?
   |RECORD VERBATIM.  PROBE FOR COMPLETE ANSWER.|

   _____ (41-43)

   _____ (44-46)

   _____ (47-49)

44c. Is there a medical doctor or osteopath (s/he) might go to if (s/he) needed
medical care?

        Yes, there is.............(50( ___ -1  (ASK Q.45a)

        No, is not.................... ___ -2 )
        Refused....................... ___ -7  \ (SKIP TO Q.46a)
        Not sure/don't know........... ___ -8  /
        No answer/interviewer error... ___ -9 )

45a.  Where does (s/he) usually go -- to a doctor's office, a clinic, a hospital, or some other place?

---

PROBE WITH A, B, OR C BEFORE RECORDING.
A.  IF CLINIC:  Is it a private clinic; a hospital outpatient clinic; a company or union clinic; a school clinic; a neighborhood or government-sponsored clinic; or any other clinic not connected with a hospital?
      IF CAN'T SPECIFY, RECORD "CLINIC" UNDER "OTHER."

B.  IF HOSPITAL:  Is it a hospital outpatient clinic or a hospital emergency room?
      IF CAN'T SPECIFY, RECORD "HOSPITAL" UNDER "OTHER."

C.  IF SOME OTHER PLACE:  What type of place is it?

---

Doctor's office or private clinic..........(51(____-1 ⎞
Company or union clinic.........................____-2 ⎟
School clinic...................................____-3 ⎬ (ASK Q.45b)
Neighborhood or government-sponsored clinic....____-4 ⎟
Hospital outpatient clinic.....................____-5 ⎟
Hospital emergency room........................____-6 ⎠

Health maintenance organization (HMO)..........____-7  (SKIP TO Q.45c)

Other place (SPECIFY)

_____ ..____-8  (ASK Q.45b)


Refused...................................(52(____-7 ⎞
Not sure/don't know...........................____-8 ⎬(SKIP TO Q.45c)
No answer/interviewer error...................____-9 ⎠


45b.  Is that place a health maintenance organization or HMO; that is, a place you go for all or most medical care, which is paid for by a fixed monthly or annual amount?

Is HMO....................(53(____-1
Isn't HMO.....................____-2
Refused.......................____-7
Not sure/don't know..........____-8
No answer/interviewer error...____-9

45c.  Is there one particular doctor (s/he) usually sees when (s/he) goes there?

Yes, is...................(54(____-1  (ASK Q.45d)

No, is not.....................____-2  
Refused........................____-7  }(SKIP TO Q.45e)  
Not sure/don't know..........____-8  
No answer/interviewer error...____-9  

45d.  What is his or her name?

_____
(RECORD NAME)

| INTERVIEWER CODE |  
Yes, doctor named...........................(55(____-1  
No, doctor not named............................____-2  
Refused.........................................____-7  
Not sure/don't know.............................____-8  
No answer/interviewer error.....................____-9  

45e.  How long has (s/he) been going to (PLACE MENTIONED IN Q.45a)?  
| DO NOT READ LIST |

Less than 1 year.........(56(____-1  
1 year but less than 2 years..____-2  
2 years.....................____-3  
3 years.....................____-4  
4 years.....................____-5  
5 years.....................____-6  
6 years or more  
SPECIFY:  WRITE IN YEARS

_____....(57-58)  
Refused.................(59)____-7  
Not sure/don't know..........____-8  
No answer/interviewer error...____-9  

| ASK EVERYONE |  
46a.  What was the month and year of (her/his) most recent medical visit -- when (s/he) actually saw a doctor in an office or at a clinic?

Month_____  Year_____

Within last 12 months............(60(____-1  (ASK Q.46b)

Longer ago (SPECIFY)

_____(61-62)  
(WRITE IN YEARS)  
Refused...........................(63(____-7 (SKIP TO Q.47)  
Not sure/don't know...................____-8  
No answer/interviewer error..........____-9

46b. To what type of place did (s/he) go for this last visit -- did (s/he) go to a doctor's office, a clinic, a hospital, or some other place?

```
PROBE WITH A, B, OR C BEFORE RECORDING.
A.  IF CLINIC:  Was it a private clinic; a hospital outpatient clinic; a company or
                union clinic; a school clinic; a neighborhood or government-sponsored
                clinic; or any other clinic not connected with a hospital?
                │IF CAN'T SPECIFY, RECORD "CLINIC" UNDER "OTHER."│

B.  IF HOSPITAL:  Was it a hospital outpatient clinic or a hospital emergency room?
                  │IF CAN'T SPECIFY, RECORD "HOSPITAL" UNDER "OTHER."│

C.  IF SOME OTHER PLACE:  What type of place was it?
```

```
        Doctor's office or private clinic..........(64(____-1⎫
        Company or union clinic.......................____-2 ⎪
        School clinic.................................____-3 ⎬(ASK Q.46c)
        Neighborhood or government-sponsored clinic...____-4 ⎪
        Hospital outpatient clinic....................____-5 ⎪
        Hospital emergency room.......................____-6⎭

        Health maintenance organization (HMO)..........____-7  (SKIP TO Q.46d)

        Other place (SPECIFY)

        _____..____-8  (ASK Q.46c)

        Refused...................................(65(____-7⎫
        Not sure/don't know...........................____-8⎬(SKIP TO Q.46d)
        No answer/interviewer error...................____-9⎭
```

46c. Was that place a health maintenance organization or HMO (that is, a place you go for all or most medical care, which is paid for by a fixed monthly or annual amount)?

```
                Was HMO..................(66(____-1
                Wasn't HMO...................____-2
                Refused......................____-7              │67-80Z│
                Not sure/don't know..........____-8
                No answer/interviewer error...____-9
```

46d. Is this the place (s/he) usually goes to for care, or not?

```
                Yes, is place usually goes.......(11(____-1  (SKIP TO Q.46f)

                No, isn't place usually goes.........____-2  (ASK Q.46e)

                Refused..............................____-7⎫
                Not sure/don't know..................____-8⎬(SKIP TO Q.46f)
                No answer/interviewer error..........____-9⎭
```

46e. Why didn't (s/he) go to the place (s/he) usually goes for medical care the last time (s/he) was sick? │DO NOT READ LIST, MULTIPLE RECORD│

```
        Couldn't get an appointment...........(12(____-1
        It cost too much for a visit..........(13(____-1
        Had no way to get there...............(14(____-1
        It was an emergency...................(15(____-1
        Need a specialist/specific service....(16(____-1
        Referred by usual source..............(17(____-1
        Other (SPECIFY)

        _____..(18(____-1

        Refused...............................(19(____-7
        Not sure/don't know.......................____-8              │20-23Z│
        No answer/interviewer error...............____-9
```

46f. During (her/his) last visit for medical care, were you completely satisfied, somewhat satisfied, or not at all satisfied with (READ EACH ITEM)?

| | | Completely Satisfied | Somewhat Satisfied | Not At All Satisfied | Refused | Not Sure/ Don't Know | No Answer/ Interviewer Error |
|---|---|---|---|---|---|---|---|
| START AT "X" | | | | | | | |
| ( ) | a. The amount of time it took (her/him) to get there.....................(24( | -1 | -2 | -3 | -7 | -8 | -9 |
| ( ) | b. The amount of time (s/he) had to wait to see the doctor, once there........(25( | -1 | -2 | -3 | -7 | -8 | -9 |
| ( ) | c. The amount of time the doctor spent with (her/him).................(26( | -1 | -2 | -3 | -7 | -8 | -9 |
| ( ) | d. The information given to you about what was wrong with (her/him), or about what was being done for (her/him).............(27( | -1 | -2 | -3 | -7 | -8 | -9 |
| ( ) | e. The out-of-pocket cost for the medical care received, that is, the cost not paid by insurance..............(28( | -1 | -2 | -3 | -7 | -8 | -9 |
| ( ) | f. The quality of the care you felt was provided at that visit.....................(29( | -1 | -2 | -3 | -7 | -8 | -9 |
| ASK ITEM "g" LAST | | | | | | | |
| | g. This visit to the doctor, overall...................(30( | -1 | -2 | -3 | -7 | -8 | -9 |

SKIP TO Q.49

47. Did (s/he) see or talk to a doctor any time during the past twelve months, that is since (DATE ONE YEAR AGO) 1981? This includes visits to the doctor and any visit to a nurse or other medical person on the doctor's staff, instead of the doctor.

Yes, saw or talked to......(31( ___-1  (SKIP TO Q.49)

No, didn't see or talk to......___-2  (ASK Q.48)

Refused........................___-7
Not sure/don't know...........___-8 } (SKIP TO Q.49)
No answer/interviewer error....___-9

48. Why hasn't (s/he) seen or spoken with a doctor in the last year?
DO NOT READ LIST -- MULTIPLE RECORD

Wasn't sick/didn't need one...................(32(   -1
Didn't know a doctor or clinic to go to......(33(   -1
Couldn't afford to go/didn't have insurance..(34(   -1
Doesn't like doctors.........................(35(   -1
Other (SPECIFY)

_____...(36(   -1
Refused.......................................(37(   -7
Not sure/don't know...........................___-8
No answer/interviewer error...................___-9

SKIP TO Q.50

49.  How many of each of the following kinds of visits did (s/he) have with a doctor or doctor's assistant during the past twelve months, that is, since (DATE ONE YEAR AGO) 1981?

| READ EACH ITEM AND RECORD NUMBER OF VISITS/CALLS.  IF "NOT SURE," RECORD "999." IF "NONE," RECORD "000." |

Number of Visits

House calls by a doctor or doctor's assistant............._____
(38-39-40)

Visits to a doctor's office or private clinic............._____
(41-42-43)

Visits to a company or union clinic......................_____
(44-45-46)

Visits to a school clinic................................_____
(47-48-49)

Visits to a neighborhood or government-sponsored clinic..._____
(50-51-52)

Visits to a hospital outpatient clinic...................._____
(53-54-55)

Visits to a hospital emergency room....................._____
(56-57-58)

Visits to any other place for medical care, other than when you may have been a patient overnight in a hospital (SPECIFY)

_____..._____
(62)                                           (59-60-61)

50.  Has (s/he) personally had a medical emergency anytime in the last year -- since (DATE ONE YEAR AGO) 1981, or not?

Yes, have had medical emergency.........(63(_____-1  (ASK Q.51a)

No, have not had medical emergency..........____-2
Refused....................................____-7  } (SKIP TO Q.54a)
Not sure/don't know........................____-8
No answer/interviewer error................____-9

|64-67Z|

-26-        CARD 10/11             824002

51a.  To what type of place did (s/he) go for emergency medical care -- to a doctor's
office, a clinic, a hospital, or some other place?
[IF MORE THAN ONE EPISODE, PROBE FOR MOST RECENT]

PROBE WITH A, B, OR C BEFORE RECORDING.
A.  IF CLINIC:   Was it a private clinic; a hospital outpatient clinic; a company or
                 union clinic; a school clinic; a neighborhood or government-sponsored
                 clinic; or any other clinic not connected with a hospital?
                 [IF CAN'T SPECIFY, RECORD "CLINIC" UNDER "OTHER."]

B.  IF HOSPITAL: Was it a hospital outpatient clinic or a hospital emergency room?
                 [IF CAN'T SPECIFY, RECORD "HOSPITAL" UNDER "OTHER."]

C.  IF SOME OTHER PLACE:  What type of place was it?

              Doctor's office or private clinic..........(68(____-1 ⎞
              Company or union clinic........................____-2 ⎟
              School clinic..................................____-3 ⎟ (ASK Q.51b)
              Neighborhood or government-sponsored clinic....____-4 ⎟
              Hospital outpatient clinic.....................____-5 ⎟
              Hospital emergency room........................____-6 ⎠

              Health maintenance organization (HMO)..........____-7  (SKIP TO Q.52a)

              Other place (SPECIFY)

              _____ ..____-8  (ASK Q.51b)

              Didn't go anywhere.............................____-9  (SKIP TO Q.54a)

              Refused....................................(69(____-7 ⎞
              Not sure/don't know............................____-8 ⎟ (SKIP TO Q.52a)
              No answer/interviewer error....................____-9 ⎠

                                                          [70-80Z]

     51b.  Was that place a health maintenance organization or HMO (that is, a place
     you go for all or most medical care, which is paid for by a fixed monthly or
     annual amount)?

                      Was HMO....................(11(____-1
                      Wasn't HMO.....................____-2
                      Refused........................____-7
                      Not sure/don't know............____-8
                      No answer/interviewer error...____-9      [12-23Z]

52a.  Did (s/he) have any problems in getting there, or not?

                      Yes, had problems..........(24(____-1  (ASK Q.52b)

                      No, didn't have problems........____-2 ⎞
                      Refused.........................____-7 ⎟ (SKIP TO Q.53)
                      Not sure/don't know.............____-8 ⎟
                      No answer/interviewer error.....____-9 ⎠

     52b.  What were the problems in getting there?  What else?

     _____  (25-26)

     _____  (27-28)

     _____  (29-30)

53. Thinking about that experience with emergency care, were you completely satisfied, somewhat satisfied, or not at all satisfied with (READ EACH ITEM)?

| START AT "X" | | Completely Satisfied | Somewhat Satisfied | Not At All Satis- fied | Re- fused | Not Sure/ Don't Know | No Answer/ Inter- viewer Error |
|---|---|---|---|---|---|---|---|
| ( ) a. | The amount of time it took (her/him) to get there..............(31( | -1 | -2 | -3 | -7 | -8 | -9 |
| ( ) b. | The amount of time (s/he) had to wait to see the doctor, once there........(32( | -1 | -2 | -3 | -7 | -8 | -9 |
| ( ) c. | The amount of time the doctor spent with (her/him)............(33( | -1 | -2 | -3 | -7 | -8 | -9 |
| ( ) d. | The information given to you about what was wrong with (her/him) or about what was being done for (her/him)............(34( | -1 | -2 | -3 | -7 | -8 | -9 |
| ( ) e. | The out-of-pocket cost of the medical care you received, that is, the cost not paid by insurance.(35( | -1 | -2 | -3 | -7 | -8 | -9 |
| ( ) f. | The quality of the care you felt was provided at that visit.............(36( | -1 | -2 | -3 | -7 | -8 | -9 |

| ASK ITEM "g" LAST | | | | | | | |
|---|---|---|---|---|---|---|---|
| g. | This visit to the doctor, overall.......(37( | -1 | -2 | -3 | -7 | -8 | -9 |

ASK EVERYONE

54a. Has (s/he) been a patient overnight in a hospital during the past twelve months, since (DATE ONE YEAR AGO) 1981?

                    Yes, has been a patient.........(38(    -1  (ASK Q.54b)

                    No, has not been a patient...........____-2 ⎫
                    Refused..............................____-7 ⎬(SKIP TO Q.56a)
                    Not sure/don't know..................____-8 ⎪
                    No answer/interviewer error..........____-9 ⎭

54b. How many times was (s/he) admitted to a hospital since (DATE ONE YEAR AGO) 1981?

                    _____Times  (39-41)
                    (RECORD NUMBER)

                    Refused...................(42(    -7
                    Not sure/don't know...........____-8
                    No answer/interviewer error...____-9

54c. Altogether, how many nights did (s/he) stay in a hospital during that period, that is since (DATE ONE YEAR AGO) 1981?

                    _____Nights  (43-45)
                    (RECORD NUMBER)

                    Refused...................(46(    -7
                    Not sure/don't know...........____-8
                    No answer/interviewer error...____-9

224  Access to Medical Care in the U.S.

55. The last time (s/he) was in the hospital overnight were you completely satisfied, somewhat satisfied, or not at all satisfied with (READ EACH ITEM)?

| START AT "X" | | Completely Satisfied | Somewhat Satisfied | Not At All Satis- fied | Re- fused | Not Sure/ Don't Know | No Answer/ Inter- viewer Error |
|---|---|---|---|---|---|---|---|
| ( ) | a. The availability of doctors whenever they were needed | (47( -1 | -2 | -3 | -7 | -8 | -9 |
| ( ) | b. The availability of nurses whenever they were needed | (48( -1 | -2 | -3 | -7 | -8 | -9 |
| ( ) | c. The out-of-pocket cost to you of the care received -- that is, the cost not paid by insurance | (49( -1 | -2 | -3 | -7 | -8 | -9 |
| ( ) | d. The information given to you about what was wrong with (her/him) or about what was being done for (her/him) | (50( -1 | -2 | -3 | -7 | -8 | -9 |
| ( ) | e. The quality of the care received from doctors in the hospital | 51( -1 | -2 | -3 | -7 | -8 | -9 |

ASK ITEM "f" LAST

| ( ) | f. The overall quality of the care you felt (s/he) got at the hospital | (52( -1 | -2 | -3 | -7 | -8 | -9 |
|---|---|---|---|---|---|---|---|

ASK EVERYONE
56a. Has (s/he) ever had (READ EACH ITEM), or not?

| | Yes, Has Had | No, Hasn't Had | Refused | Not Sure/ Don't Know | No Answer/ Inter- viewer Error |
|---|---|---|---|---|---|
| a. A skin test or any kind of test for tuberculosis or TB | (53( -1 | -2 | -7 | -8 | -9 |
| b. An injection or shot against measles | (54( -1 | -2 | -7 | -8 | -9 |
| c. DPT or baby shots, that is, injections against diphtheria, whooping cough, or tetanus | (55( -1 | -2 | -7 | -8 | -9 |
| d. A shot or medicine against polio | (56( -1 | -2 | -7 | -8 | -9 |
| e. A hearing test | (57( -1 | -2 | -7 | -8 | -9 |

56b. In the last twelve months, has (s/he) (READ EACH ITEM), or not?

| | Yes, Has | No, Hasn't | Refused | Not Sure/ Don't Know | No Answer/ Inter- viewer Error |
|---|---|---|---|---|---|
| a. Had an eye examination | (58( -1 | -2 | -7 | -8 | -9 |
| b. Been treated or examined by a dentist | (59( -1 | -2 | -7 | -8 | -9 |

-29-    CARD 11    824002

57a.  Does (s/he) go to school during the school year, or not?

          Goes to school............(60(    -1
          Does not go to school.........____-2
          Refused.....................____-7
          Not sure/don't know..........____-8
          No answer/interviewer error...____-9

ASK Q.58 IF PROXY IS CHILD'S MOTHER AND CHILD IS UNDER 4.  IF CHILD IS 4 OR OVER, OR
PROXY NOT MOTHER, SKIP TO INSTRUCTIONS AT END OF INTERVIEW.

58.  Thinking back to your pregnancy before (s/he) was born, how many months pregnant
were you when you started seeing a doctor about the pregnancy regularly?

          1 month or less...........(61(    -1
          2.............................____-2
          3.............................____-3
          4.............................____-4
          5.............................____-5
          6.............................____-6
          7.............................____-7
          8.............................____-8
          9.............................____-9
          Refused...................(62(____-7
          Not sure/don't know...........____-8
          No answer/interviewer error...____-9

IF ADULT OR ADULT PROXY INTERVIEW NOT ALREADY COMPLETED, GO TO FACTUALS, AND SET UP
APPOINTMENT TIME FOR ADULT INTERVIEW.

IF ADULT INTERVIEW AND FACTUALS ALREADY COMPLETED, THANK AND TERMINATE.

Time at this Point: _____ : _____ o'clock  AM..(67(____-1
                    (63-64)   (65-66)           PM......____-2

68-80Z

# Index

# Center for Health Administration Studies
## Graduate School of Business
## Division of Biological Sciences
## The University of Chicago
## Research Series

RS #1 — *The Behavioral Scientists and Research in the Health Field — a questionnaire survey*, Odin W. Anderson, Ph.D., and Milvoy Seacat. 1957. 15 pp.

RS #2 — *An Examination of the Concept of Medical Indigence*, Odin W. Anderson, Ph.D., and Harold Alksne. 1957. 14 pp.

RS #3 — *The Prescription Pharmacist Today*, Wallace Croatman and Paul B. Sheatsley. 1958. 27 pp.

RS #4 — *The Public Looks at Hospitals*, Eliot Freidson and Jacob J. Feldman. 1958. 24 pp.

RS #5 — *Public Attitudes Toward Health Insurance*, Eliot Freidson and Jacob J. Feldman. 1958. 18 pp.

RS #6 — *The Public Looks at Dental Care*, Eliot Freidson and Jacob J. Feldman. 1958. 16 pp.

RS #8 — *Health Research Opportunities in Welfare Records — a preliminary report on illness and economic dependency*, Herbert Notkin, M.D., M.P.H. 1958. 20 pp.

RS #9 — *Comprehensive Medical Insurance — a study of costs, use, and attitudes under two plans*, Odin W. Anderson, Ph.D., and Paul B. Sheatsley. 1959. 105 pp.

RS #11 — *Measuring Health Levels in the United States, 1900–1958*, Odin W. Anderson, Ph.D., and Monroe Lerner. 1960. 38 pp.

RS #12 — *An Examination of the Concept of Preventive Medicine*, Odin W. Anderson, Ph.D., and George Rosen, M.D., Ph.D., 1960. 22 pp.

RS #13 — *Hospital Use and Charges by Diagnostic Category — a report on the Indiana study of a Blue Cross population*, Monroe Lerner. 1960. 32 pp.

RS #18 — *Proprietary Nursing Homes — a report on interviews with 35 nursing home operators in Detroit, Michigan*, Thomas E. Mahaffey. 1961. 44 pp.

RS #19 — *Hospital Use by Diagnosis — a comparison of two experiences*, Monroe Lerner. 1961. 46 pp.

RS #21 — *An Analysis of Personnel in Medical Sociology*, Odin W. Anderson, Ph.D., and Milvoy S. Seacat. 1962. 8 pp.

RS #22 — *Syphilis and Society — problems of control in the United States, 1912—1964*, Odin W. Anderson, Ph.D. 1965. 62 pp.

RS #23—*People and Their Hospital Insurance—comparisons of the uninsured, those with one policy, and those with multiple coverage*, Ronald Andersen and Donald C. Riedel, Ph.D. 1967. 37 pp.

RS #24—*Hospital Use—a survey of patient and physician decisions*, Odin W. Anderson, Ph.D., and Paul B. Sheatsley. 1967. 215 pp.

RS #25—*A Behavioral Model of Families' Use of Health Services*, Ronald Andersen, Ph.D. 1968. 106 pp.

RS #26—*Health Services in the Chicago Area, a framework for use of data*, Odin W. Anderson, Ph.D., and Joanna Kravits. 1968. 133 pp.

RS #27—*Medical Care Use in Sweden and the United States*, Ronald Andersen, Ph.D., Björn Smedby, Med. Lic., and Odin W. Anderson, Ph.D. 1970. 174 pp.

RS #28—*The Relationship Between Administrative Activities and Hospital Performance*, Duncan Neuhauser, Ph.D. 1971. 115 pp.

RS #29—*Ambulatory Use of Physicians' Services in Response to Illness Episodes in a Low-Income Neighborhood*, William C. Richardson, Ph.D. 185 pp.

RS #30—*Patterns of Dental Service Utilization in the United States: A Nationwide Social Survey*, John F. Newman, Ph.D., and Odin W. Anderson, Ph.D. 127 pp.

RS #31—*A Model of Physician Referral Behavior: A Test of Exchange Theory in Medical Practice*, Stephen Shortell, Ph.D. 200 pp.

RS #32—*Access to Medical Care in the U.S.: Who Has It, Who Doesn't*, Lu Ann Aday, Ph.D., Gretchen V. Fleming, Ph.D., Ronald M. Andersen, Ph.D. 1984.

RS #33—*HMO Development: Patterns and Prospects*, Odin W. Anderson, Ph.D., Terry E. Herold, A.M., Bruce Butler, M.B.A., Claire Kohrman, M.A., Ellen M. Morrison, M.A. 1984.

A price list and copies of RS #1 through #31 can be obtained directly from the Center for Health Administration Studies, University of Chicago, 1101 East 58th Street, Chicago, IL 60637. RS #32 and #33 can be purchased through Pluribus Press, Inc., 160 East Illinois Street, Chicago, IL 60611.